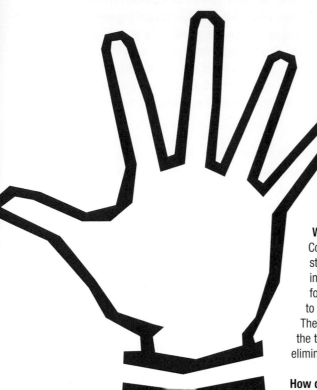

Tips on how to use this book
This workbook has several special features that make it easier to access and use the material.

How do I find a particular subject?
A general table of contents is shown on p.5. The first page of each chapter gives detailed information on its contents, and numbered color tabs on the right edge of the page make it easy to locate a particular page or chapter. You can also use the subject index at the end of the book. For added clarity, key words and phrases of special interest are highlighted in the text.

What about anatomic orientation?
Complex image planes are matched with explanatory diagrams that identify key structures. The numbers in the diagrams appear in bold type in the accompanying text on the same page (no annoying page flipping), or you can refer to the fold-out number key on the back flap of the book. The numbers in the key apply to all the diagrams in the book.

The directions of arrow symbols used in illustrations always match the arrows in the text. Two arrows pointing in the same direction never appear on the same page, eliminating confusion.

How do I find a particular illustration?
Very simple: all the figures and tables are numbered by the page on which they appear. For example, **Fig. 99.2** is on p. 99.

How do I remember all the normal values, formulas, and percentages?
No need. All this information is printed on sturdy, washable, pocket-sized reference cards at the back of the book. Simply cut them out and carry them with you.

Can I test my knowledge and review essential points?
Each chapter ends with a critical evaluation comparing color duplex with alternative modalities, followed by a self-test quiz with review questions and images. By taking the quiz, you can test your progress and identify areas that need further review.

How do the diagrams work?
Particular types of tissue are shown in the same gray levels and colors throughout the book:

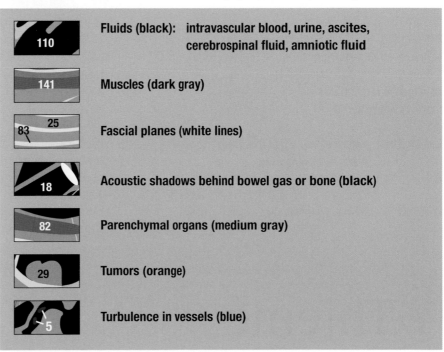

110	**Fluids (black):** intravascular blood, urine, ascites, cerebrospinal fluid, amniotic fluid
141	**Muscles (dark gray)**
83 \ 25	**Fascial planes (white lines)**
18	**Acoustic shadows behind bowel gas or bone (black)**
82	**Parenchymal organs (medium gray)**
29	**Tumors (orange)**
5	**Turbulence in vessels (blue)**

Matthias Hofer, M.D., MPH, MME (Editor)
Institute for Diagnostic Radiology
(Head: U. Mödder, M. D.)
Heinrich-Heine University
P.O. Box 10 10 07
40001 Düsseldorf,
Germany

List of authors see p. 4

Important Note: Medicine is an ever-changing science undergoing continual development. Research and clinical experience are continually expanding our knowledge, in particular our knowledge of proper treatment and drug therapy. Insofar as this book mentions any dosage or application, readers may rest assured that the authors, editors, and publishers have made every effort to ensure that such references are in accordance with the state of konwledge at the time of production of the book.

Nevertheless this does not involve, imply, or express any guarantee or responsibility on the part of the publishers in respect of any dosage instructions and forms of application stated in the book. Every user is requested to examine carefully the manufacturers' leaflets accompanying each drug and to check, if necessary in consultation with a physician or specialist, whether the dosage schedules mentioned therein or the contraindications stated by the manufacturers differ from the statements made in the present book. Such examination is particularly important with drugs that are either rarely used or have been newly released on the market. Every dosage schedule or every form of application used is entirely at the user's own risk and responsibility. The authors and publishers request every user to report to the publishers any discrepancies or inaccuracies noticed. If errors in this work are found after publication, errata will be posted at www.thieme.com on the product description page.

© 2010 Georg Thieme Verlag,
Rüdigerstraße 14, 70469 Stuttgart, Germany
http://www.thieme.de
Thieme New York, 333 Seventh Avenue,
New York, N.Y. 10001 USA
http://www.thieme.com

Designed by   Inger Wollziefer, Bonn, Germany
                 www.designinger.de
Printed in Germany by
                 Druckerei Steinmeier, Nördlingen, Germany
Photos by   Markus Meuthen, Düsseldorf, Germany

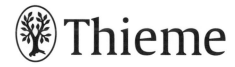

ISBN 978-3-13-127593-6

Matthias Hofer's Color Duplex Sonography is an excellent example of a compact yet all encompassing textbook. As in his other books, Dr. Hofer has created an exceptionally well-organized text that begins with an overview of the principies of color Doppler imaging and proceeds to the application of this important modality throughout the body. The richly illustrated chapters demonstrate the usefulness of color duplex ultrasound not only in vascular disease, but also in the evaluation of multiple organ systems in the neck, thorax, abdomen, and pelvis. Each chapter begins with normal anatomy shown with color and power Doppler images of extraordinary quality that are well labeled and matched with line drawings. The application of color duplex ultrasound in detecting and characterizing various disease states is then laid out with concise descriptions and beautiful images. This book is a fine introduction to color duplex ultrasound imaging and is a welcome addition to the sonographic literature.

Arnost Fronek, M.D., Ph.D.
Prof. of Surgery and Bioengineering
Dept. of Surgery
University of California, San Diego, USA

Abbreviations used

α	alpha = insonation angle	ECA	external carotid artery	PDV	peak diastolic velocity
AAA	abdominal aortic aneurysm	ECG	electrocardiography	PHA	proper hepatic artery
AAPG	arm-ankle pressure gradient	ED	end-diastolic	PI	pulsatility index
ABI	ankle-brachial index	EDA	end-diastolic area	PRF	pulse repetition frequency
ACA	anterior cerebral artery	EP	ectopic pregnancy	PSV	peak systolic velocity
AIUM	American Institute for Ultrasound in Medicine (Bioeffects Committee)	ES	end-systolic	PTA	percutaneous transluminal angioplasty
		ESA	end-systolic area		
		F_0	transmitted frequency	PV	portal vein
A_N	area of normal vessel lumen	FAC	fractional area change	PW	pulsed wave, pulsed Doppler
A_0	aorta	F_E	frequency of returning echoes	RA	right atrium
A_S	area of intrastenotic residual lumen	FFTS	fetofetal transfusion syndrome	RAS	renal artery stenosis
		FNH	focal nodular hyperplasia	RI	resistance index
ASD	atrial septal defect	FS	fractional shortening	RT	renal transplant
A-SMA	automatic segmental motion analysis	HCC	hepatocellular carcinoma	RV	right ventricle
		HPRF	high pulse repetition frequency	RVOT	right ventricular outflow tract
AT	acceleration time	HVs	hepatic veins	SA	splenic artery
AV	atrioventricular	ICA	internal carotid artery	SCC	squamous cell carcinoma
AV fistula	arteriovenous fistula	ICS	intercostal space	S_i	segmental area
AVM	arteriovenous malformation	IMA	inferior mesenteric artery	SMA	superior mesenteric artery
ß-HCG	human chorionic gonadotropin	IUGR	intrauterine growth retardation	SMV	superior mesenteric vein
B mode	brightness-modulated ultrasound image (gray-scale)	IVF	in vitro fertilization	SV	sample volume, stroke volume
		LA	left atrium	T_E	echo delay time
CCA	common carotid artery	LN	lymph node	TEE	transesophageal echocardiography
CDS	color duplex scanning (sonography)	LV	left ventricle		
		LVOT	left ventricular outflow tract	THI	tissue harmonic imaging
CHA	common hepatic artery	M mode	motion mode (series of B-mode dots displayed over time)	TIA	transient ischemic attack
CIV	common iliac vein			TIPSS	transjugular intrahepatic portosystemic shunt
CO	cardiac output				
CSAR	cross-sectional area reduction	M/T ratio	ratio of maximum diameter to transverse diameter	T_{SV}	transit time through the SV
CT	computed tomography			UA	umbilical artery
CTG	cardiotocography	MCA	middle cerebral artery	UV	umbilical vein
CVI	chronic venous insufficiency	MCL	midclavicular line	V	blood flow velocity
CW	continuous-wave Doppler	MHz	megahertz (1 million cycles per second)	V_{max}	peak systolic velocity (= PSV)
dB	decibel			VOD	veno-occlusive disease
DICOM	Digital Imaging and Communications in Medicine	MRA	magnetic resonance angiography	VSD	ventricular septal defect
		MRI	magnetic resonance imaging	VTI	velocity-time integral
DPI	Doppler perfusion index	PAOD	peripheral arterial occlusive disease		
DSA	digital subtraction angiography				
DVT	deep vein thrombosis (in the lower extremity)	PCA	posterior cerebral artery		

Institute of Diagnostic Radiology
(Director: Prof. U. Mödder, M.D.)
Heinrich Heine University
Moorenstrasse 5, 40225 Düsseldorf
Germany

Matthias Hofer, M.D., MPH, MME (Editor)
Andreas Saleh, M.D.
Marco Pieper

Department of Diagnostic and
Interventional Radiology
(Director: Prof. Michael Forsting, M.D.)
University Hospital Essen
Hufelandstr. 55, 54122 Essen
Germany

Prof. Gerald Antoch, M.D.

Vitos Clinic of Neurology Weilmünster GmbH
Weilstraße 10, 35789 Weilmünster
Germany

Andreas Dietz, M.D.

Department of Nephrology and Rheumatology
Knappschafts-Hospital
Osterfelder-Str. 155a, 46242 Bottrop
Germany

Markus Hollenbeck, M.D., Ph.D.

Pediatric Cardiology and CHD
Heart Center Duisburg
Gerrickstr. 21, 47137 Duisburg
Germany

Otto N. Krogmann, M.D., Ph.D.

Department of Obstetrics and Gynecology
(Director: Prof. Wolfgang Janni, M.D.)
Heinrich Heine University
Moorenstrasse 5, 40225 Düsseldorf
Germany

Tatjana Reihs, M.D.

Head of Department of Neurology
Klinikum Herford
Schwarzmoorstrasse 70, 32049 Herford
Germany

Prof. Matthias Sitzer, M.D.

Department of Neurology
University Hospital Zurich
Frauenklinikstrasse 26, CH - 8091 Zurich
Switzerland

Ghazaleh Tabatabai, M.D., Ph.D.

Contents

Q

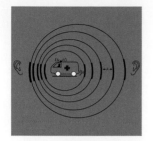

Matthias Hofer

Introduction

This workbook is for sonographers who already have experience with gray-scale B-mode ultrasound imaging and would like to learn more about color Doppler ultrasound (CDU) or echocardiography. Therefore, we will not be covering the basic principles of B-mode imaging and common artifacts as it is assumed that the reader already knows about these or can review them by consulting a basic textbook of ultrasonography (see inside front cover).

This chapter deals with the basic principles that are important for understanding color flow imaging, time-varying Doppler spectra, and possible sources of error. The chapter also presents guidelines on choosing the best equipment settings for a particular application.

The principles and sample applications of technical innovations in CDU are presented at the end of the book. Take the quiz starting on p. 112 to test your knowledge of ultrasound fundamentals before proceeding with the organ-specific applications of CDU.

Basic physical and technical principles

Piezoelectric effect

When an alternating voltage is applied to ceramic elements, known in clinical parlance as "crystals", the elements will change their shape in proportion to the cyclic alternation of the electric current. This sets up pressure waves with a frequency in the range of several megahertz, above the range of human hearing.

Conversely, sound waves that return to the transducer as echoes cause the crystals to vibrate, inducing an electric voltage that can be processed to generate an ultrasound image.

Principle of Doppler ultrasound

The basis for determining the velocity and direction of blood flow is the Doppler effect, discovered by the physicist Christian Johann Doppler in 1842. This effect states that when a sound source and a reflector are moving toward each other, the sound waves are spaced closer together and reach the receiver at a higher frequency (F_E) than they were originally emitted (F_0). This is the same effect responsible for the apparent rising pitch of an approaching ambulance siren (**Fig.8.3a**) and the falling pitch as the ambulance moves away (**Fig. 8.3b**).

Effect of beam angle

If we apply this phenomenon to red cells moving through blood vessels, additional factors come into play. The magnitude of the frequency shift (ΔF) is proportional not only to the blood flow velocity (**V**) and the original transmitted frequency (**F0**), but also to the speed of sound in human tissue (**C**) and the angle of the ultrasound beam (α) relative to the long axis of the vessel (**Fig.8.2**). The examiner must always measure this angle in order to obtain accurate velocity information. Because sound waves travel through human tissue at a relatively constant speed of approximately 1540 m/s and the other factors in the Doppler equation (**Table 8.1**) are also predefined, the frequency shift depends strongly on the cosine of the beam-vessel angle. In the least favorable case, where the beam is angled 90° to the vessel axis (**Fig.8.5**), the frequency shift equals zero – i.e., no signal is detected even when flow is present.

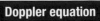

Doppler equation
$$\Delta F = F_E - F_0 = 2 \times F_0 \times \frac{V}{C} \times \cos\alpha$$
F_E = Frequency of echo
F_0 = Transmitted frequency
V = Blood flow velocity
C = Speed of sound in human tissue (approximately 1540 m/s)
a = Beam-vessel angle

Table 8.1

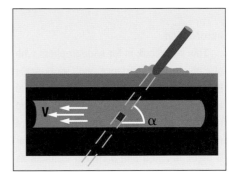

Fig. 8.2

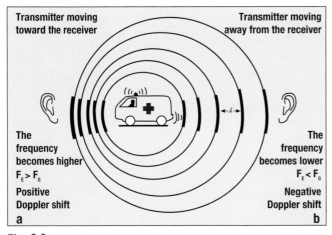

Fig. 8.3

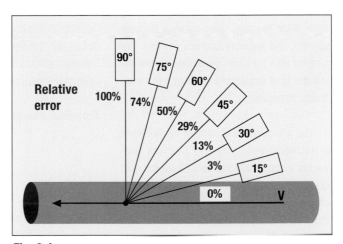

Fig. 8.4

The most favorable case with the smallest error would be a beam – vessel angle of 0° – i.e., a beam directed precisely along the vessel axis. The more closely the angle approaches 90°, the greater the relative error (**Fig. 8.4**). Consequently, the beam should be angled no more than 60° to the vessel axis, and an angle of 45° or less is even better. A Doppler angle in this range can minimize errors in the flow velocity, which is calculated in cm/s from ΔF and α.

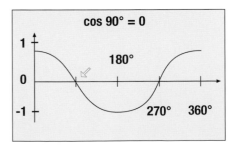

Fig. 8.5

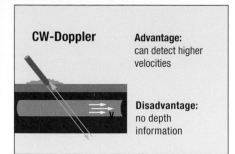

Fig. 9.1

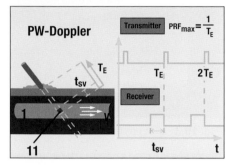

Fig. 9.2

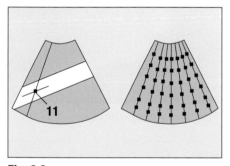

Fig. 9.3

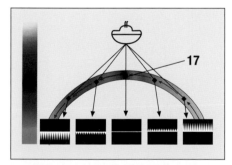

Fig. 9.4

Function of different Doppler techniques

In continuous-wave (CW) Doppler **(Fig.9.1)**, the sound beam is continuously emitted from one piezoelectric crystal and received by a separate crystal. The advantage of CW is its ability to detect and record even very high frequency shifts. The disadvantage is its insensitivity to the depth of the echo source.

In pulsed-wave (PW) Doppler **(Fig.9.2)**, the sound beam is alternately transmitted and received using only one crystal. The echo delay time **(T_E)** can be converted to distance, and so the depth of the echo source can be determined. This is necessary in order to construct a two-dimensional color duplex image **(Fig. 9.3)**, in which gray-scale B-mode ultrasound is combined with numerous PW sample volumes **(11)** to generate a two-dimensional image. The smaller the color box (the image area selected for color encoding), the faster a new image can be generated and the higher the temporal resolution.

The number of pulses that are transmitted per second is called the pulse repetition frequency **(PRF)**. The PRF can be increased only to a value of $1/T_E$. It declines as scanning depth increases, as more time is needed **(TSV)** for the echoes to return from a more deeply positioned sample volume. This sets an upper limit to the flow velocities that can be accurately recorded with pulsed Doppler. As a result, vessels with higher flow velocities must be examined with a higher PRF setting, while slow venous flow requires a lower PRF.

Color flow

Flow directed toward the transducer is generally encoded in red, while flow away from the transducer is encoded in blue. The velocity of the flow is represented by the shade or brightness of the color: faster velocities are displayed in brighter colors. This relationship is important in the evaluation of intrastenotic flow acceleration (see p.36) and when acoustic conditions are poor (see p.38). Flow in a curved vessel may be encoded red in one segment and blue in the adjacent segment, depending on the flow direction relative to the transducer **(Fig. 9.4)**. Color brightness also varies locally in accordance with changes in the beam-vessel angle (α) (see p.8). The 90° beam angle at the junction of the red and blue segments results in a color void **(17)**, which should not be misinterpreted as a partially occlusive thrombus.

The examiner should be aware, however, that the color assignment in commercial duplex machines can be inverted at the touch of a button. The current color scheme is usually indicated on a color scale displayed at the edge of the screen: the colors in the upper half of the scale encode flow toward the transducer, and those in the lower half encode flow away from the transducer **(Fig. 9.4)**.

When a linear-array transducer is used, changing the angle of the Doppler waves by beam steering can cause the same vascular segment to be encoded in red or blue, as desired **(Fig. 9.5a)**. Angling the color box **(16)** can correct for an unfavorable beam-vessel angle, making vascular segments that initially show poor color flow **(Fig. 9.5b)** easier to evaluate **(Fig. 9.5c)**. Alternatively, the examiner can manually angle the probe on the skin to insonate the vessel at an oblique angle.

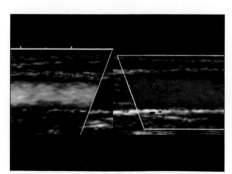

Fig. 9.5a

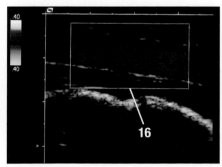

Fig. 9.5b

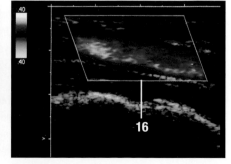

Fig. 9.5c

Interpretation of spectral waveforms

Doppler spectra are sampled from blood vessels by switching the machine to pulsed Doppler (pulsed wave, PW) **(Fig. 10.1)** and using a trackball **(Fig. 10.2)** to position the sample volume **(11)** at the center of the vessel lumen **(1)** **(Fig. 10.3)**. The frequency shifts (Δ**F**, y axis) between the emitted ultrasound pulse and the returning echo are measured in kilohertz (kHz), and the magnitude of the frequency shifts is plotted over time (x axis) and displayed as a waveform. Δ**F** is proportional to the blood flow velocity in the insonated vascular segment. However, the insonation angle must be entered before the frequency data can be converted to a "true flow velocity" (see pp. 8, 17).

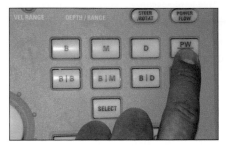

Fig. 10.1 Activating PW Doppler

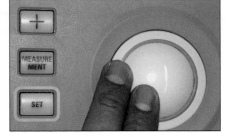

Fig. 10.2 A trackball is used …

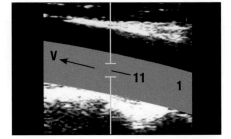

Fig. 10.3 … to position the sample volume

For each point in time at which signals are acquired, the scanner calculates and displays a velocity distribution consisting of slower and faster flow components **(Fig. 10.4)**. **Figure 10.5** illustrates a typical waveform recorded from a central artery. When the systolic pulse wave arrives at the Doppler sampling site, the flow velocity (V) rises sharply from slow or zero flow at end diastole to the maximum flow velocity **(V$_{max}$)**, which is also called the peak systolic velocity **(PSV)** (⇩). Note the almost vertical upstroke of the systolic peak (⇲ in **Fig. 10.5**), showing that very little time passes (time to peak, **TTP**) from the start of systole until the peak velocity **(12)** is reached. A delay in the upstroke (⟺), resulting in a more oblique waveform with a prolonged TTP **(Fig. 10.6)**, is suggestive of stenosis proximal to the sampling site. The stenosis may be located in the sampled vessel itself or in a more proximal feeding artery (see p. 14).

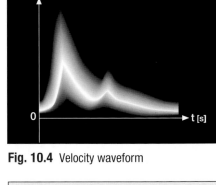

Fig. 10.4 Velocity waveform

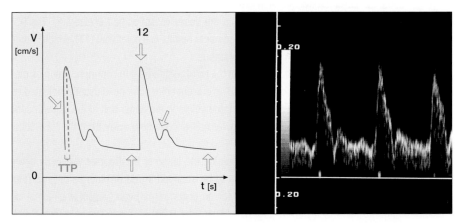

Fig. 10.5 Normal spectral waveform from central arteries

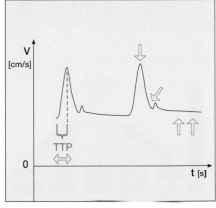

Fig. 10.6 Waveform distal to a stenosis

Biphasic waveform in central arteries

Arteries near the heart normally pump blood against a relatively low peripheral resistance, resulting in a biphasic waveform. Blood flows from the heart to the periphery (cardiofugal flow) throughout the cardiac cycle. The flow is always directed forward at a velocity that is higher in systole than in diastole. The smaller end-diastolic velocity peak is generally separated from the systolic peak by a small notch (⬚) caused by closure of the aortic valve.

The lower the momentary resistance of the downstream vessels, the higher the level of the (end-) diastolic flow (⇧). Thus, an elevated diastolic waveform (⇧⇧) may mean that the perfusion demand of the peripheral structures supplied by that artery is increased as a result of exercise, or it may signify a pathologic decrease in blood flow (ischemia) **(Fig. 10.6)**.

Triphasic waveform in peripheral arteries

At greater distances from the heart, blood vessels increasingly lose their expansion-chamber or windkessel function while the peripheral resistance at the Doppler sampling site increases. As a result, the peripheral arteries exhibit a "triphasic" waveform composed of three distinct phases: Systole is again characterized by rapid cardiofugal flow toward the periphery. Generally this upstroke falls off rapidly, as in the more central vessels, and often terminates in a small notch (✑) caused by closure of the aortic valve.

Due to the higher resistance in the peripheral arteries, early diastole is normally marked by a brief period of reverse flow (**13**, ↗) directed back toward the heart (cardiopetal, 2nd phase), appearing as a deflection below the baseline. This downstroke introduces a negative value into the calculated Doppler indices (see p. 12). It is followed by a small upstroke that again indicates flow toward the periphery (3rd phase, **Fig. 11.1**). End diastole may show zero flow (⇓) caused by high peripheral resistance (e.g., at rest or during cold-induced vasoconstriction) or may demonstrate slow cardiofugal flow. The latter is more likely to occur at higher ambient temperatures or when there is mild to moderate exertion of the muscles supplied by the artery.

More vigorous muscular exercise stimulates the release of vasodilator messengers that lower the peripheral resistance until the reverse flow component disappears. Since the curve no longer dips below the baseline, the previously triphasic waveform changes physiologically to a biphasic waveform with an increased PSV (↘) and an elevated level of diastolic flow (⇑⇑) (**Fig. 11.2**).

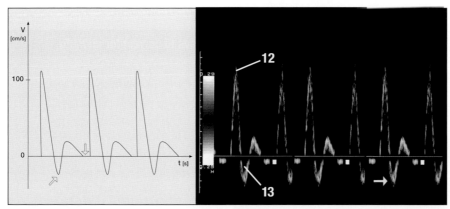

Fig. 11.1 Normal spectral waveform from peripheral arteries

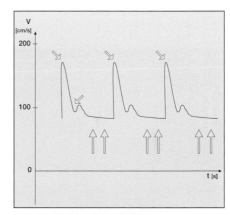

Fig. 11.2 Waveform change in response to exercise

At rest, the physiologic boundary between the two waveform patterns is located in the aorta at the origin of the renal arteries, each of which supplies an organ with low flow resistance. The higher flow resistance of the pelvic and lower extremity muscles often prevails below that level, causing a triphasic waveform to develop in the distal abdominal aorta.

Stress tests

Stress tests can illustrate how rapidly the vascular system adapts to the increased demand caused by exercise. The iliofemoral arteries, for example, can be tested by having the patient lie supine and carry out rapidly alternating dorsiflexion and plantarflexion of the ankle joint for approximately 30-45 seconds or make circling movements of the foot at the ankle and subtalar joints. The upper extremity arteries can be tested in a similar fashion by having the patient rapidly open and close the fist during Doppler scanning. Normally, the waveform changes rapidly from a triphasic pattern at rest to a biphasic pattern during exercise and then changes swiftly back again, showing <u>no</u> evidence of stenosis at or proximal to the sampling site (see pp. 13/14).

Doppler indices

The **PSV**, the mean flow velocity (**V$_{mean}$**), and the diastolic velocity (**V$_{diast}$**) are used to calculate indices for evaluating arterial flow that are **in**dependent of the beam-vessel angle **(Table 12.1)**. These indices are not distorted by imprecise or incorrect angle data. They have proved particularly useful for evaluating small and short arteries within the renal parenchyma, for example, to aid in the early detection of allograft rejection (see pp. 51-55).

Pulsatility index (PI) of Gosling
$$PI = \dfrac{V_{peak} - V_{diast}}{V_{mean}}$$

Resistance index (RI) of Pourcelot
$$RI = \dfrac{V_{peak} - V_{diast}}{V_{peak}}$$

Table 12.1

Aliasing

If the measured frequency shift exceeds the Nyquist limit of the pulse repetition frequency (PRF)/2 at very high flow velocities, the corresponding portion of the waveform will be cut off and displayed on the opposite side of the spectrum **(Fig. 12.2a)**. This phenomenon is analogous to the "wagon wheel" effect in Western movies, in which the wheel spokes suddenly appear to rotate in the opposite direction due to the slow frame rate of the film. Aliasing in Doppler spectra can be corrected by increasing the PRF or shifting the zero baseline **(Fig. 12.2b)**.

Aliasing in the color flow image is manifested by color reversal at the center of the vessel marked by a predominance of bright spectral colors. This may occur, for example, in vessels with intra- or poststenotic flow acceleration or if the PFR has been set too low **(Fig. 12.3a)**. **Figure 12.3b** shows the same image following adjustment of the PRF. This phenomenon differs from a true reverse flow component, in which the darker areas of the color spectrum predominate. Other ways to correct for aliasing are listed in **Table 12.4**.

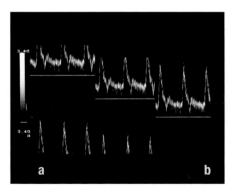

Fig. 12.2 Aliasing in the Doppler spectrum

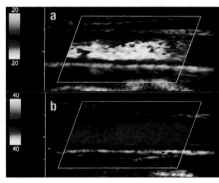

Fig. 12.3 Aliasing in the color flow image

Ways to correct for aliasing
• Increase the PRF. If the PRF is already on maximum:
• Decrease the penetration depth
• Shift the baseline (can double the range of measurable frequencies)
• Use a lower-frequency transducer
• Increase the insonation angle α (within limits, as this will increase the range of error)

Table 12.4 Compensating for aliasing

General hemodynamic theory

When a large vessel bifurcates, the previously laminar flow pattern (⬇) increasingly assumes a parabolic shape (⬇) reflecting a greater difference between the higher flow velocities at the center of the lumen and the slower flow along the vessel wall **(Fig. 12.5)**.

If fat pads or calcifications cause the normally smooth vessel wall to become irregular, this will disturb the laminar flow pattern and give rise to turbulent zones (see **Fig. 13.3**).

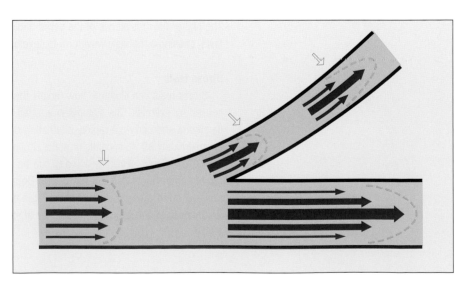

Fig.12.5

Signs of stenosis in the Doppler spectrum

These signs depend not only on the degree of stenosis but also on the location of the sampling site relative to the stenosis. When the ultrasound probe is placed proximal to an arterial stenosis, the sampled waveform is quite different from that recorded within the stenosis or at varying distances beyond it.

A waveform acquired proximal to a stenosis will often show little or no change, depending on the availability of collateral vessels **(Fig. 13.1)**. But a waveform recorded a short distance proximal to the stenosis, with no intervening arteries that can function as collaterals, will typically show a "backwash" pattern, especially at sites just proximal to a very-high-grade (subtotal) stenosis or occlusion. When the pulse wave encounters a vascular occlusion and is reflected back from it, the spectrum shows an abnormal increase in reverse flow with very little delay in the TTP and little decrease in the PSV **(Fig. 13.2)**.

The reverse flow component (displayed here below the baseline) lasts longer (⟺) than the systolic inflow (displayed here above the baseline), but it reaches only about one-third (⇑) or one-fourth of the peak systolic velocity, depending on the wall elasticity of the affected vascular segment. As a result, the shaded areas bounded by the waveform deflections above and below the baseline are of approximately equal size. Thus, for example, while a carotid artery occlusion at the skull base or in the carotid siphon generally cannot be detected directly, finding an associated backwash pattern in the ipsilateral internal carotid artery (ICA) can be very helpful in further diagnosis or planning treatment.

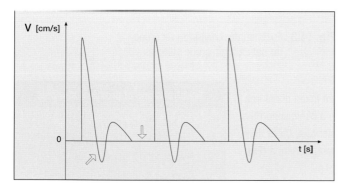

Fig. 13.1 Prestenotic waveform often shows no changes

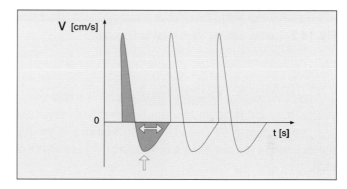

Fig. 13.2 Waveform proximal to an occlusion

By contrast, an intrastenotic waveform shows a very definite increase in flow velocity. The smaller the residual lumen of the artery, the faster the blood must travel through the site of narrowing, with a corresponding increase in V_{max} or PSV. With a relatively high-grade stenosis (>75% luminal narrowing), the intrastenotic flow acceleration **(15a)** may reach values of several meters per second. This acceleration is still detectable for several centimeters past the stenosis as a "poststenotic jet" **(15b)** but falls off rapidly with increasing distance from the stenosis **(Fig. 13.3)**. Unlike a "normal" waveform, the intrastenotic waveform recorded from a subtotal stenosis no longer returns to slow velocities but remains high, interrupted only by systolic peaks (⬋) spiking above the elevated waveform **(Fig. 13.4)**.

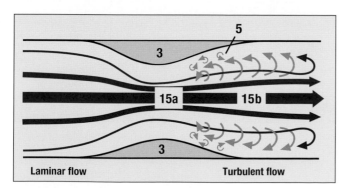

Fig. 13.3 Intrastenotic flow acceleration with turbulent zones near the vessel wall **(5)**

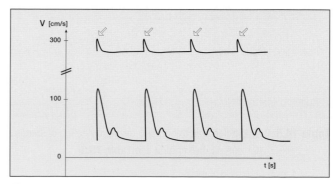

Fig. 13.4 Waveform recorded in a high-grade stenosis >90% (above) compared with a normal waveform (below).

Because this intrastenotic flow acceleration generally increases in proportion to the degree of luminal narrowing, the intrastenotic PSV can serve as a measure for the degree of stenosis (see **Table 78.3**). The PSV ratio, which relates the intrastenotic PSV to the pre- or poststenotic PSV of the same arterial segment, has proved to be a useful measure for the quantification of multiple consecutive stenoses [1.7]. This ratio **(Table 14.1)** ensures that the estimated degree of stenosis is not distorted by the presence of other, adjacent stenoses.

Another criterion for stenosis in intrastenotic or immediate poststenotic waveforms is filling in of the spectral window **(12)** below the systolic peak. This means that turbulence at the time of the PSV has also given rise to unusually slow velocity components **(Fig. 14.2a)** which normally should not exist in laminar flow – at least at the center of the vessel during systole **(Fig. 14.2b)**.

Quantification of stenosis with the PSV ratio	
PSV-ratio	Reduction in cross-sectional area
< 2.5	0 - 49 %
> 2.5	50 - 74 %
> 5.5	75 - 99 %

Table 14.1

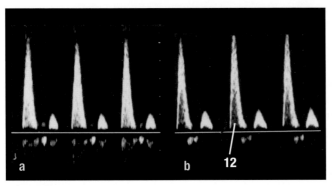

Fig. 14.2 Spectral window: filled in (**a**) and clear (**b**)

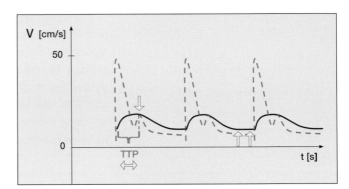

Fig. 14.3 Poststenotic waveform recorded far past a high-grade stenosis

A spectrum acquired far past the stenosis, such as a tibial artery spectrum taken distal to a stenosis of the ipsilateral femoral artery, is marked by a delayed upstroke to a diminished PSV (⇓) and a prolonged TTP (⇔) (see p. 10). Depending on the degree of stenosis, there may also be a relative elevation of diastolic velocities (⇑) as evidence of peripheral ischemia **(Fig. 14.3)**.

Spectral signs of proximal stenosis
1) Poststenotic decrease in PSV (depends on degree of collateralization)
2) Poststenotic lengthening of TTP
3) Poststenotic elevation of diastolic waveform (depends on degree of ischemia)

Table 14.4

Taken all criteria for stenotic arterial disease together, we can observe the following signs **(Table 14.5)**:

Criterion	Sampling site			
	prestenotic	intrastenotic	poststenotic jet	far poststenotic
PSV	normal	⇑ - ⇑⇑	(⇑)	⇓
TTP	normal	normal	(⇑)	⇑
Level of diastolic flow	normal or possible increase in reverse flow	normal - ⇑⇑ (depending on degree of stenosis)	⇑	⇑ - ⇑⇑ (depending on degree of stenosis)
Spectral window	clear	(may be filled in)	filled in	normal

Table 14.5 Qualitative spectral criteria for the detection of stenosis (for quantitative criteria see **Table 78.3**)

Eleven steps to an optimum image

The steps that are necessary to obtain a flawless, optimized B-mode image, color flow image, and Doppler spectrum are summarized in **Table 15.1** and detailed below. This table is also included on the removable checklist page so that it can be cut out and carried in your labcoat pocket.

Steps of Image Optimization	
B-mode image	
Step 1	Angle the probe relative to the vessel axis
Step 2	Place just one focal zone at the center of the vessel lumen
Step 3	Set the B-mode gain to a low level
Color flow image	
Step 4	Use beam steering to improve the beam-vessel angle (angled away from 90°, see p. 8)
Step 5	Adjust the PRF to the prevailing flow velocity
Step 6	Increase the color gain until blooming occurs, then lower the gain until color signals are confined to the vessel lumen (no extravascular color pixels)
Doppler spectrum	
Step 7	Position the sample volume (SV) at the center of the vessel and set the SV size at $^1/_2$ to $^2/_3$ of the luminal diameter
Step 8	Adjust the baseline level for spectral components above or below the baseline to eliminate waveform cutoff at the top or bottom
Step 9	Adjust the velocity range (PRF_{PW}). If aliasing still occurs: Doppler trace too short => $PRF_{PW}\downarrow$ => to expand the trace vertically Doppler trace too high => $PRF_{PW}\uparrow$ => to compress the trace vertically
Step 10	Adjust the PW gain to obtain a good contrast-to-noise ratio: Try to get a dark background without noise pixels, but do not set the gain too low (for automatic envelope curve detection)
Step 11	Remember to enter the insonation angle!

Table 15.1

Optimizing the B-mode image

The ultrasound probe should be angled slightly ( ) so that the ultrasound wavefront will strike the vessel wall obliquely and not at a 90° angle **(Fig. 15.2)**. This is especially important for scanning vessels that run parallel to the skin, such as the carotid arteries. Care is taken to maintain acoustic contact with the skin ( ) when angling the probe. The next step is to position a single focal zone at the depth corresponding to the center of the vessel **(Fig. 15.3)**, since multiple focal zones will often cause too much slowing of the frame rate. The final step is to reduce the B-mode gain slightly ("a little too dark") to improve the quality of subsequent color flow imaging **(Fig. 15.4)**. Generally this is done by either turning a dial counterclockwise ( ) or lowering a slide switch.

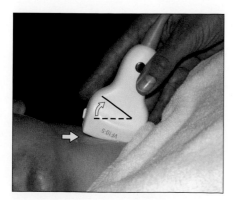

Fig. 15.2 Angling the probe

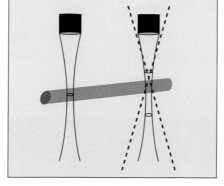

Fig. 15.3 One focal zone is placed at the center of the vessel

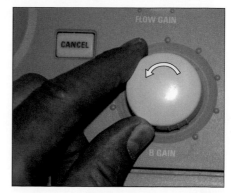

Fig. 15.4 Lowering the gain

Optimizing the color flow image

Step 4: When using a linear probe, you can improve the insonation angle (see **Fig. 8.4**) by activating beam steering to angle the ultrasound wavefront relative to the vessel of interest. This is done by pushing a "steer" button one or more times **(Fig. 16.1)** or by turning a dial, depending on the machine and the manufacturer. This should significantly improve color encoding, especially at the edges of the vessel **(Fig. 16.2)**, compared with regular settings **(Fig. 16.3)**.

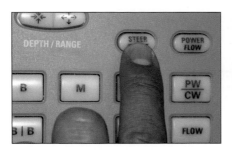

Fig. 16.1 Beam steering angulation

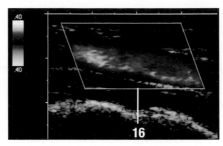

Fig. 16.2 With beam steering

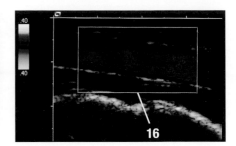

Fig. 16.3 Without beam steering

Step 5: Optimize the color illumination of the vessel lumen by adjusting the PRF to the prevailing velocity. If a color reversal **(6)** occurs during systole with a predominance of bright spectral colors (aliasing, see p. 12) **(Fig. 16.4)**, incrementally adjust the PRF or velocity switch to increase the PRF (in arteries, by just one step per pulse length) until the aliasing just disappears **(Fig. 16.5)**.

If initial aliasing does not occur during systole, or if color voids appear in the peripheral part of the vessel lumen **(17)** **(Fig. 16.6)**, lower the PRF incrementally until color reversal occurs, then set the PRF just one step higher. Do not mistake color reversal caused by "true" backflow (with a predominance of dark = low-velocity spectral colors) for aliasing.

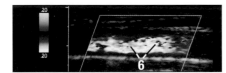

Fig. 16.4 PRF too low => aliasing

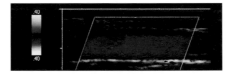

Fig. 16.5 Optimum PRF setting

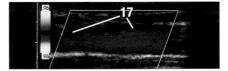

Fig. 16.6 PRF is too high

Step 6: The last step in color adjustment is to optimize the color gain. Check if the color pixels are superimposed over the intima-media echo in an artery or over the edge of a venous vessel ("blooming" artifact), and check for any extravascular color signals **(Fig. 16.7)**. Blooming indicates excessive color gain that would hamper the detection of any thrombi that may be adherent to the vessel wall.

If the gain is set too high, turn the color gain control counterclockwise (or lower the slide switch) just to the point at which blooming disappears **(Fig. 16.8)**.

Conversely, if the initial image shows incomplete color filling of the vessel lumen **(Fig. 16.9)**, turn the color gain dial clockwise (or raise the slide switch) until blooming just appears in systole, then reduce the gain slightly.

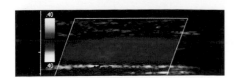

Fig. 16.7 Blooming artifact

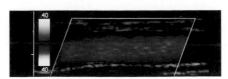

Fig. 16.8 Optimum color gain

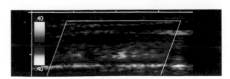

Fig. 16.9 Color gain is too low

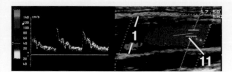

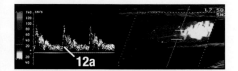

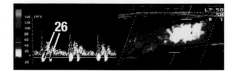

Fig. 17.1 SV in correct position

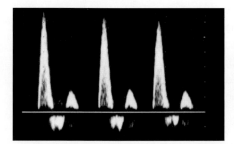

Fig. 17.2 SV off-centered

Fig. 17.3 SV too large

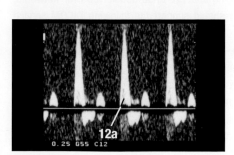

Fig. 17.4 Adjusting the zero baseline

Optimizing the Doppler spectrum

Step 7: On most machines, pulsed Doppler is activated by pressing the PW or D button. This automatically displays a sample volume (SV, **11**) at the center of the image. Position the sample volume at the center of the vessel lumen **(1)**, then adjust its size to $1/2$ or at most $2/3$ of the vessel diameter **(Fig. 17.1)**.

If the SV is positioned off-center near the edge of the vessel, it will also detect low-velocity components, causing the previously clear spectral window (**12a** in **Fig. 17.2**) to fill in relative to the normal setting **(Fig. 17.1)**. This loss of the clear spectral window could be mistaken for turbulence, creating a false-positive sign of stenosis.

This effect is compounded by making the SV too large, so that it not only detects slow flow velocities near the vessel wall but also detects wall movements due to vascular pulsations. These movements will appear in the Doppler spectrum as bright artifacts **(26)** located near the baseline **(Fig. 17.3)**.

Step 8: If portions of the spectrum appear clipped, you can correct this by shifting the baseline. With a biphasic or venous waveform, this will display the spectrum on just one side of the baseline **(Fig. 17.4)**. With a triphasic waveform, the level of the baseline should be adjusted so that approximately $2/3$ to $3/4$ of the image height is displayed on the systolic side and only $1/4$ to $1/3$ on the side with the reverse flow component.

Step 9: If the spectrum is still clipped vertically relative to a normal setting **(Fig. 17.5)** despite adjustment of the baseline **(Fig. 17.6)**, the velocity range (PRF$_{PW}$) should be increased in order to compress the Doppler trace. If the trace appears too short **(Fig. 17.7)**, you can expand it vertically by reducing the PRF$_{PW}$.

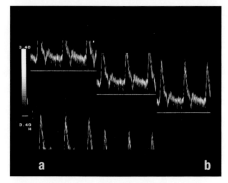

Fig. 17.5 PRF$_{PW}$ is correct

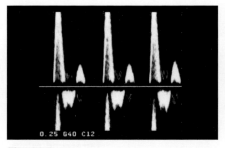

Fig. 17.6 PRF$_{PW}$ is too low

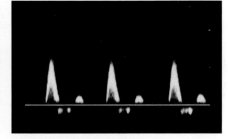

Fig. 17.7 PRF$_{PW}$ is too high

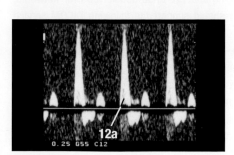

Fig. 17.8 PW gain is too high

Step 10: Now adjust the amplification of the Doppler signal (PW gain) to display the waveform at maximum intensity while just eliminating unwanted background noise (pixels outside the "true" spectral trace). Otherwise, the subsequent use of automatic peak-velocity envelope curve detection will yield false values or time will be lost adjusting the sensitivity for the detection program. Excessive Doppler gain may also cause spurious filling in **(12a)** of the spectral window **(Fig. 17.8)**.

Step 11: Finally, do not forget to enter the insonation angle so that the machine will display accurate velocity information in cm/s (see p. 8).

Common sources of error		
Problem	**Cause**	**Solution**
Low signal amplitudes or poor color encoding	Beam angle > 60°	Use more oblique probe angle
	B-mode gain too high	Reduce B-mode gain
	Color gain too low	Increase color signal gain
	PRF too high (in veins)	Decrease PRF
	Wall filter too high (in veins)	Reduce color wall filter
Aliasing despite normal B-mode and pulsed Doppler	PRF too low	Increase PRF or shift the baseline
Low velocities despite normal color image	Faulty angle correction	Realign the angle correct bar parallel to the vessel axes
Spectral window in pulsed Doppler fills in with normal audio signal and flow velocities	PW gain too high	Reduce PW gain until the background appears black (free of noise)
Doppler trace from peripheral arteries shows normal triphasic pattern but is above the baseline	Hyperemia after physical exertion, causing decrease in peripheral resistance	Rest the patient at least 10 min and repeat the examination

Table 18.1

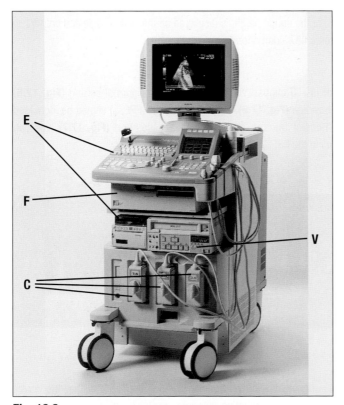

Fig. 18.2

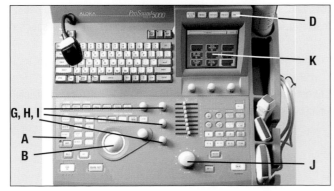

Fig. 18.3

Equipment requirements

A high-capacity scan converter **(A)** is advantageous for nearly all applications. A trackball **(B)** can be used to access and retrieve the optimum point in the cardiac cycle from the cine-loop memory. Three separate plug-in ports **(C)** enable the user to switch between different transducers at the touch of a button **(D)**, eliminating the need to plug and unplug transducer cords during the examination. Digital image archiving **(E)** and communication over data networks have become DICOM-compliant on some machines **(Fig. 18.2)**, although with some manufacturers you should still give this feature a practical test before purchasing the device (see below). The system should include a color printer **(F)** and video recorder **(V)** to make findings available for outpatients and third parties. The controls for PRF **(G)**, color gain **(H)**, pulsed Doppler gain **(I)**, and B-mode gain **(J)** are shown in **Figure 18.3**. Another useful feature is the ability to store several user-defined settings **(K)**, eliminating the need to adjust all the parameters for each examination.

Ultrasound-relevant DICOM requirements

If color duplex imaging data are to be transferred over networks, the ultrasound system should support the following DICOM service classes:

- Storage (network-compliant single-image and cine-loop storage in gray scale and color)
- Print (print functions for gray scale and color)
- Worklist management (transfer of patient data from hospital information system)
- Media storage (on removable media)
- Structured reporting.

The system should support supplements 1, 2, 3, 5, 10, 29, and 31.

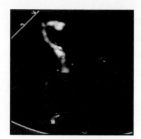

Andreas Dietz
Matthias Hofer
Matthias Sitzer

Introduction

The main goal of cerebrovascular imaging with CDS is to quantify the degree of stenosis caused by atherosclerotic vascular disease in symptomatic patients who have a history of transient ischemic attacks or completed stroke. The study should establish both the degree of stenosis and the length of the affected vascular segment. The collateral circulation should also be assessed to determine the preoperative or preinterventional complication risk. An accurate study requires a knowledge of cerebrovascular anatomy and normal findings, which will be reviewed in this chapter before turning to typical vascular lesions affecting the anterior and posterior circulations.

Cerebrovascular anatomy

First, look at the diagram on the left and see if you can name the numbered blood vessels. If there are some you cannot identify, check the numbers that are boldfaced in the text below.

The circle of Willis is normally supplied by the carotid arteries **(anterior circulation)** and the vertebral arteries (posterior circulation). The origin of the common carotid artery (CCA, **40**) from the aortic arch **(30e)** on the right side and from the brachiocephalic trunk **(115)** on the left side are relatively infrequent sites of plaque formation. Stenoses most commonly develop at the site where the CCA bifurcates into the internal carotid artery (ICA, **40a**) and the external carotid artery (ECA, **40b**). The first intracranial branch of the ICA is the ophthalmic artery. Just beyond it, the ICA divides into the middle cerebral artery (MCA, **54b**) and the anterior cerebral artery (ACA, **54a**) **(Fig. 19.1)**.

The **posterior circulation** is supplied by the vertebral arteries **(55)**. In about 4% of cases they spring directly from the aortic arch **(30e)**, but usually they arise from the subclavian artery **(116)**, often arising at a more proximal level on the left side than on the right. Each vertebral artery is subdivided into five segments **(Table 19.2)**. The proximal segment near the origin is called V_0. The V_1 segment usually extends to the transverse process of the C_6 vertebra, but occasionally the artery enters the foramen at the C_5 level. The V_2 segment is most accessible to ultrasound examination midway up the neck. The atlas loop of the vertebral artery constitutes the V_3 segment. The V_4 segment is intracranial, and the posterior inferior cerebellar artery (PICA, **55a**) arises from its distal portion. The vertebral artery may be hypoplastic in certain segments or throughout its course. The right and left vertebral arteries unite to form the basilar artery **(56)**, which branches into the posterior cerebral artery **(54c)** on each side.

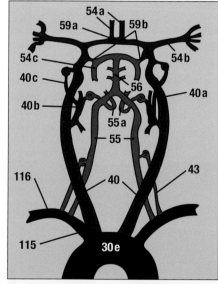

Fig. 19.1

**Segmental anatomy
of the vertebral arteries**

V_0: Origin from the subclavian artery
V_1: From V0 to entry into transverse foramina
V_2: Segment within the costotransverse canal (C_2 - C_6)
V_3: Segment at the level of the atlas loop
V_4: Terminal intracranial segment

Table 19.2

Collateral pathways

1. Severe stenosis or occlusion of the ICA: In the principal collateral pathway from the ECA **(40b)** to the anterior territory of the ICA **(40a)**, blood enters the skull by a retrograde route via the supratrochlear artery **(164a)** and ophthalmic artery **(164)** **(Fig. 20.1)**. Alternatively, the contralateral ICA can compensate for a high-grade stenosis by supplying crossover flow through the anterior communicating artery **(59a)** **(Fig.19.1)**. The surgeon must be aware of any hypoplasia or aplasia of the proximal A_1 segment in order to assess the surgical risk. Finally, the posterior circulation can supply collateral flow via the posterior communicating artery **(59b)** if the ipsilateral P_1 segment is not aplastic.

2. Severe stenosis or occlusion of the vertebral artery: A proximal vertebral artery stenosis may be collateralized by the deep cervical artery from the thyrocervical trunk **(43)** or by branches of the occipital artery **(40c)** from the ECA territory **(Fig.19.1)**. With a basilar artery stenosis, the posterior communicating arteries **(59b)** or leptomeningeal anastomoses from the MCA territory form the only available collateral channels. Aplasia of the P_1 segment with a direct origin of the PCA from the ICA can have a beneficial effect in such cases.

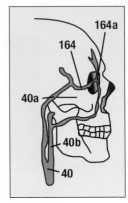

Fig. 20.1

Normal findings in the anterior circulation

Many examiners prefer to assume a sitting position behind the head of the recumbent patient **(Fig. 20.2a)**. Scanning can also be initiated from the front by placing the transducer next to the midline and visualizing the CCA **(40)** in transverse section **(Fig. 20.2b)**. Generally, this vessel is located posteromedial to the internal jugular vein **(41a)**. Normal respiratory variations in the caliber of the jugular vein can be accentuated by having the patient perform a Valsalva maneuver; often this permits immediate identification of the vessel in the B-mode image. Normally the transverse plane is displayed as if viewed from below, causing an apparent reversal of right and left.

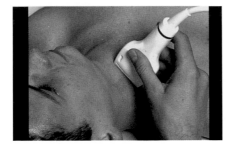

Fig. 20.2a

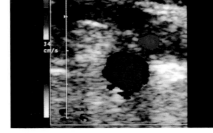

Fig. 20.2b

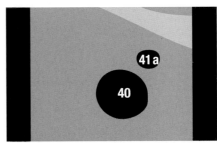

Fig. 20.2c

When the transducer is rotated 90° to the longitudinal axis **(Fig. 20.3a)**, the right side of the image is inferior and the left side is superior, as in abdominal ultrasound [2.1]. Watch for the physiologic flow separation **(7)** that occurs where the CCA bifurcates and widens into the carotid bulb on the side of the ICA **(40a, Fig. 20.3b)**. This abrupt expansion normally creates a circumscribed vortex, which should not be mistaken for pathologic poststenotic flow reversal, turbulence, or aliasing.

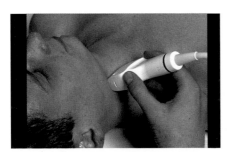

Fig. 20.3a

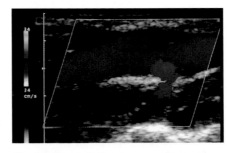

Fig. 20.3b

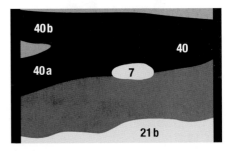

Fig. 20.3c

The Doppler spectrum of the CCA **(Fig. 20.4)** usually shows a somewhat higher peak systolic velocity (PSV) than the ICA. The ICA **(Fig. 20.5)** shows a higher level of diastolic flow (⇓) due to the relatively low intracranial peripheral resistance. This contrasts with the ECA **(40b)**, which typically produces a "swishing" audio signal with relatively high systolic velocities and low diastolic velocities. The ECA may show a triphasic spectrum that includes a reverse flow component (↖) **(Fig. 20.6)**. Here the superior thyroid artery **(43a)** is visible in the color display.

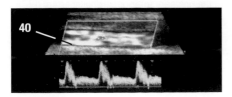

Fig. 20.4

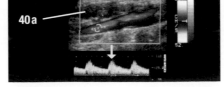

Fig. 20.5

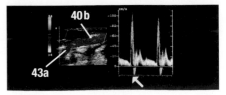

Fig. 20.6

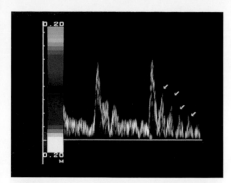

Fig. 21.1

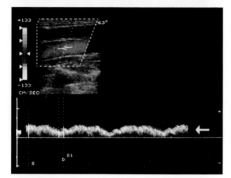

Fig. 21.2

Anatomic orientation

When imaged in the long axis, the ICA normally runs posterolaterally, moving away from the transducer, while the ECA remains close to the transducer over a longer distance. If vessel identity is in doubt, repetitive compression of the superficial temporal artery will produce an oscillation (✎) of the ECA spectral waveform **(Fig. 21.1)**. The internal jugular vein **(41a)** is easily distinguished from the ICA by its flow direction (⇐) and its flat spectral trace **(Fig. 21.2)**.

Stenotic lesions of the internal carotid arteries

Atherosclerotic deposits do not always contain shadowing calcifications. "Soft plaques" (✎) **(3)** appear as hypoechoic, crescent-shaped or circumferential voids in the color-filled lumen **(1)** along the vessel wall **(Fig. 21.3a)**. The craniocaudal extent (↖ ↗) of the plaque can be accurately documented with CDS **(Fig. 21.3b)**. **Figure 21.4a** shows a higher-grade, calcified ICA stenosis **(10)** with intrastenotic and poststenotic turbulence **(5)** and an acoustic shadow **(18)**. The residual lumen **(1)** is often defined more clearly in the power Doppler mode (see p. 106) **(Fig. 21.4b)**. It is also common to find eccentric flow acceleration **(15a)**, in this case by 290 cm/s. Aliasing **(6)** (color shift from yellow to green) is present on the vessel wall opposite the plaque **(Fig. 21.5)**. In the case of an occlusion **(22)**, even the most sensitive color-flow setting will show only hypoechoic plaque **(4)** in place of the intraluminal flow signal **(Fig. 21.6)**. The display shows an ICA occlusion in longitudinal section **(a)** and transverse section **(b)** with the adjacent ECA **(40b)** and a typical occlusion signal **(c)** with an absence of end-diastolic flow (⇓). The flow reversal in the vascular stump produces a characteristic color pattern caused by flow hitting the obstruction in systole and reversing in diastole.

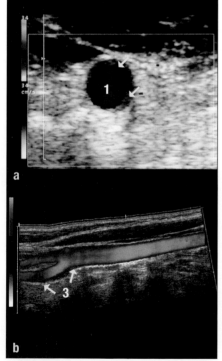

Fig. 21.3

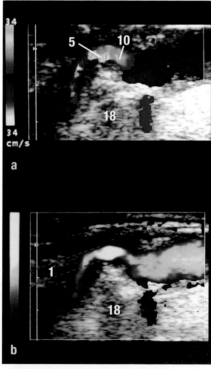

Fig. 21.4

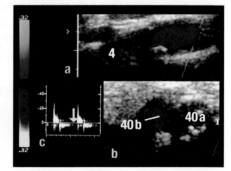

Fig. 21.5

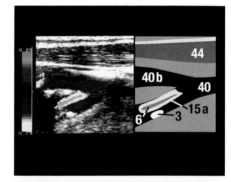

Fig. 21.6

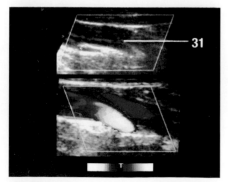

Fig. 21.7

Dissection of the vessel wall

A dissection membrane **(31)** with blood between the vessel wall layers **(Fig. 21.7)** is a special condition that is usually spontaneous but may result from a neck injury or athletic activity at any age. It is characterized by the formation of a hypoechoic, intramural hematoma that causes significant flow disturbance.

A mural aneurysm occasionally develops as a complication. The intimal flap may occlude the primary vascular channel, which tapers gradually to a sharp point in the ultrasound image. Recanalization may occur over a period of weeks and can be accurately documented with CDS.

Quantifying internal carotid stenosis

The local degree of stenosis can be calculated in a transverse image by measuring the cross-sectional area of the intrastenotic, color-filled residual lumen (A_S) and relating it to the original vascular cross section at the site of the disease (A_N) **(Fig. 22.1)** using the formula for cross-sectional area reduction (CSAR) in **Figure 22.2**. The more sensitive power Doppler mode is often better for making an accurate determination of cross-sectional area in the residual perfused lumen **(Fig. 22.3)**.

In both of the images shown, the hypoechoic intraluminal plaque **(4)** is clearly distinguishable from hyperechoic calcifications **(3)**.

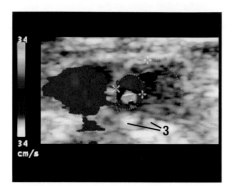

Fig. 22.1

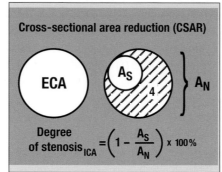

Cross-sectional area reduction (CSAR)

$$\text{Degree of stenosis}_{ICA} = \left(1 - \frac{A_S}{A_N}\right) \times 100\%$$

Fig. 22.2

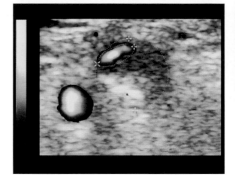

Fig. 22.3

The degree of stenosis can also be assessed in a longitudinal scan by measuring the angle-corrected peak systolic flow velocities **(Fig. 22.4)**. Intra-arterial DSA, by contrast, does not provide flow velocity data or cross-sectional images. The method used in the largest multicenter study to date (**N**orth **A**merican **S**ymptomatic **C**arotid **E**ndarterectomy **T**rial: **NASCET**) measured carotid stenosis by relating the luminal diameter at the narrowest part of the stenosis (d_S) to the normal width of the ICA distal to the stenosis (d_{ICA}) [2.2].

Regarding the use of CDS for evaluating stenosis, it has been shown that this technique can predict the angiographic degree of stenosis with a high degree of accuracy. **Table 22.5** reviews the spectral features that are associated with various grades of stenosis [2.3, 2.4]. To plan appropriate treatment, it is important to differentiate a preocclusive "pseudo-occlusion" from a complete occlusion. A filiform residual lumen that is not visible on unenhanced images can sometimes be identified after the intravenous administration of a contrast agent (see p.107) [2.5, 2.6]. It should be noted that a higher **PSV** may be detected after delivery of the intravenous contrast **(Fig. 22.6)**. CDS is also excellent for the noninvasive follow-up of carotid thromboendarterectomy (TEA) or stent implantation (✍ ✍) to exclude recurrent stenosis **(Fig. 22.7)**. Several multicenter studies have shown that carotid TEA can reduce the individual stroke risk in patients with a symptomatic high-grade stenosis (>70%) of the ICA [2.7].

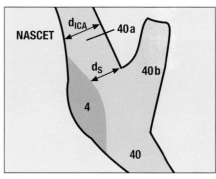

Fig. 22.4

Internal carotid stenosis					
Criteria: % stenosis	Intrastenotic PSV	Intrastenotic ΔF	Intrastenotic spectrum	Poststenotic spectrum	Flow reversal in ophthalmic artery?
< 40 % (not stenotic by definition)	< 120 cm/s	< 4 KHz	Normal	Normal	No
40 - 50 % (mild)	~ 120 cm/s	~ 4 KHz	Slight	Normal broadening	No
51 - 70 % (moderate)	~ 200 cm/s	4 - 7 KHz	Broadening	PSV ↓ V_{diast} ↑	No
71 - 90 % (high-grade)	~ 300 cm/s	> 7 KHz	Reverse flow components	PSV ↓ V_{diast} ↑	Flow ↓, zero flow or flow reversal
91 - 99 % (preocclusive)	Variable	Variable	Amplitude ↓	Variable	Frequent

Table 22.5

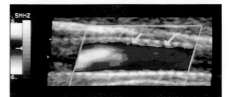

Fig. 22.6

Fig. 22.7

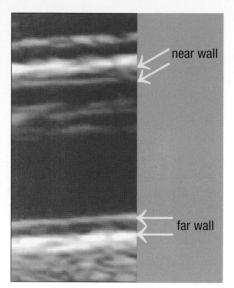

Fig. 23.1

Intima-media thickness (IMT) of the carotid system

Long-term epidemiologic studies have shown convincingly that the carotid artery intima-media thickness (IMT) is an independent predictor of subsequent stroke or myocardial infarction after adjustment for traditional risk factors (hypercholesterolemia, arterial hypertension, smoking, etc.) [2.9-2.13]. How is the IMT determined?

The technical requirements include a > 7.5-MHz linear transducer, image recording at 60-dB log compression, and vascular measurement in systole. No harmonic components or artificial contrast enhancers should be used. Starting from the carotid lumen, the first layer that can be defined sonographically is the echogenic blood-intimal interface, followed by the hypoechoic intima-medial interface, and finally the echogenic media-adventitial interface. For physical reasons, the carotid IMT can be measured much more accurately in the far wall (⇐) than in the near wall (⬈), where the interfaces are less clearly defined **(Fig. 23.1)**. The far-wall IMT is generally measured as the combined thickness of the intima-media complex, since taking separate measurements of the intima and media would not yield a valid result.

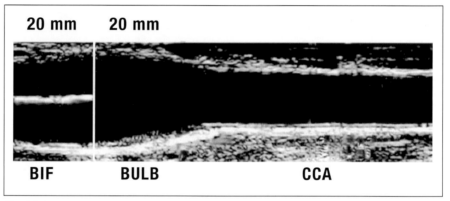

Fig. 23.2

The usual practice in scientific studies is to take 5 to 10 separate measurements in three carotid segments the CCA, carotid bifurcation, and carotid bulb and calculate a mean value for all three segments **(Fig. 23.2)**. These studies often employ semiautomatic imaging processing modules that continuously register numerous IMT values using a gray-scale process, greatly increasing the reproducibility of the measurements **(Fig. 23.3)**.

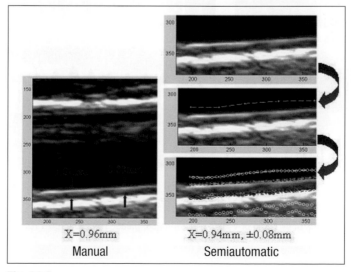

Fig. 23.3

Age (years) Male	Left CCA			Right ACC		
	50th perc.	75th perc.	95th perc.	50th perc.	75th perc.	95th perc.
< 35	0.61	0.67	0.78	0.59	0.66	0.75
35-44	0.67	0.74	0.86	0.64	0.71	0.85
45-54	0.72	0.81	1.03	0.68	0.75	0.96
55-64	0.77	0.89	1.15	0.74	0.84	1.05
65-74	0.86	0.96	1.39	0.85	0.95	1.20
≥ 75	0.91	1.05	2.17	0.88	1.01	1.85
Female	50th perc.	75th perc.	95th perc.	50th perc.	75th perc.	95th perc.
< 35	0.59	0.65	0.72	0.58	0.63	0.73
35-44	0.64	0.69	0.80	0.63	0.68	0.78
45-54	0.69	0.75	0.90	0.66	0.73	0.86
55-64	0.74	0.83	1.02	0.71	0.80	0.97
65-74	0.81	0.91	1.14	0.80	0.87	1.04
≥ 75	0.85	0.99	1.28	0.82	0.91	1.16

Table 24.1 IMT-values for CCA-measurements [2.14]

For the practical application of this test outside of scientific studies, it is convenient to limit the measurements to the CCA. One protocol consists of locating a representative segment 10 mm long, performing 5 to 10 separate measurements, and then taking the mean value. The resulting IMT values for the CCA are age-dependent (see **Table 24.1**) and correlate with established vascular risk factors (see above). The values in the table are based on 7000 screening examinations in patients at various centers with no prior history of neurologic disease [2.14] and thus constitute a representative sample of the normal German population. The 50th, 75th, and 95th percentiles are shown. **Figure 24.2** contrasts an abnormal IMT in a man approximately 50 years of age **(a)** with a normal IMT **(b)**. Interestingly, it was found in the study that the effective treatment of cardiovascular risk factors could decrease the IMT over a one- to two-year period.

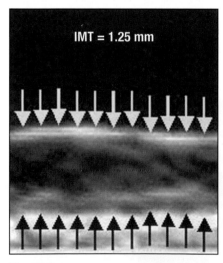

IMT = 1.25 mm

IMT = 0.67 mm

Fig. 24.2a   **Fig. 24.2b**

For automated measurements of IMT and of vessel wall stiffness, please refer to page 110.

Posterior circulation

The vertebral artery (55) is scanned in longitudinal section from the anterolateral aspect in the supine patient, starting from the vertebral artery origin (V_0) and proceeding to a point just before the atlas loop (including V_2, see p.19) (**Fig. 25.1a**). It is best to use a variable-frequency linear-array transducer operating at frequencies of 5.0-7.5 MHz. The intraforaminal V_2 segment is most accessible to duplex examination. Along with the accompanying vein (55b), this segment can be clearly visualized between the acoustic shadows (18) of the cervical vertebral bodies (21b) (**Fig. 25.1b**).

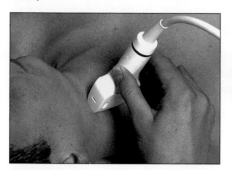

Fig. 25.1a

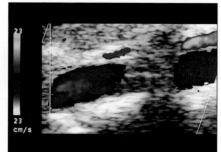

Fig. 25.1b

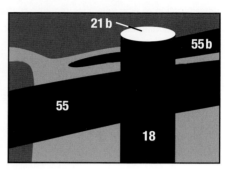

Fig. 25.1c

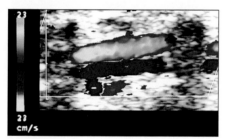

Fig. 25.2

In the most common pattern of vertebral artery hypoplasia (**Fig. 25.2**), one vertebral artery (usually the right) is less than 2.5 mm in diameter while the contralateral artery is enlarged to more than 4 mm in diameter (right-left discrepancy more than 1 : 1.7) [2.4]. The normal vertebral artery diameter is approximately 3.8 + 0.5 mm [2.8]. Hypoplastic vertebral arteries show a marked reduction in the end-diastolic flow component (V_{diast}). It is difficult to distinguish vertebral hypoplasia from distal stenosis or occlusion, both of which are associated with a reduction in Vdiast. The origin of the vertebral artery (55) from the subclavian artery (116, **Fig. 25.3**) is a site of predilection for stenosis. Another common site is the atlas loop area (**Fig. 25.4b**), which is scanned from the posterior aspect below the mastoid process. It is best to use a 5.0-MHz transducer placed just below and behind the mastoid and angled toward the contralateral orbit with the head turned slightly to the opposite side (**Fig. 25.4a**).

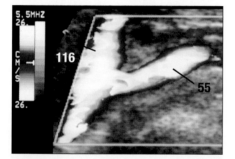

Fig. 25.3

The V4 segment is scanned transnuchally with a 2.5-MHz or 2.0-MHz sector probe (**Fig. 25.5a**). The probe is applied below the occipital protuberance and angled toward the orbit. The junction of the vertebral arteries (55) at the basilar artery (56) is shown in **Figure 25.5b**.

The spectral features of artery stenosis in general are described on pp. 13 and 78. The origin of the vertebral artery (V_0-segment) is the predilection site for the development of extracranial vertebral artery stenosis. To determine the degree of luminal narrowing, optimal cutoff values of the maximum peak systolic velocity and the peak systolic velocity ratio of the vertebral origin (V_0) versus the intravertebral segment (V_2) have been determined as well (**Table 25.6**) [2.15].

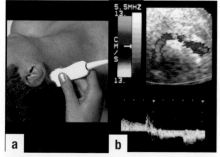

Fig. 25.4

The normal vertebral artery (**Fig. 25.7a**) exhibits a biphasic spectrum with a clear spectral window (↖), whereas stenosis is characterized by marked flow acceleration (⇒) with fill-in of the spectral window. **Figure 25.7 b** illustrates a high-grade stenosis of the V_4 segment of the left vertebral artery at its junction with the basilar artery in a woman with left-sided hemiataxia in the setting of a TIA.

Dissection of the vertebral artery following neck trauma can lead to embolic cerebral ischemia culminating in stroke. The color duplex findings can range from intramural hematoma to occlusion of the affected arterial segment. The intimal flap itself can occasionally be visualized.

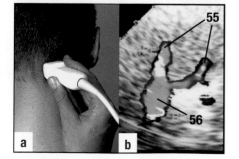

Fig. 25.5

Stenotic degree	Intrastenotic PSV	PSV-ratio of V_0 / V_2
< 50 %	≥ 85 cm/s	≥ 1.3
50-69 %	≥ 140 cm/s	≥ 2.1
70-99 %	≥ 210 cm/s	≥ 4.0

Table 25.6 Cut-off values vertebral artery

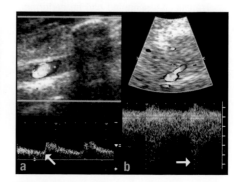

Fig. 25.7

Transtemporal examination of intracranial arteries

The thin squamous portion of the temporal bone provides the best acoustic window for scanning the circle of Willis with a 2.0-MHz transducer **(Fig. 26.1a)**. The axial scan in **Figure 26.1b+c** demonstrates the right middle cerebral artery (MCA, **54b**), the anterior cerebral artery (ACA, **54a**), the distal terminal portion of the ICA **(40a)**, the posterior communicating artery **(59b)**, and the posterior cerebral arteries (PCA, **54c**). Both the P_1 and P_2 segments of the right PCA can be identified.

The normal Doppler spectrum of the MCA **(Fig. 26.3)** shows a low-resistance pattern with correspondingly high diastolic flow (⇓). An accurate determination of flow velocities requires scanning a long vascular segment to allow for proper angle correction. Usually this can be done in the MCA by scanning along the vessel at an acute angle. This is more difficult with the PCA and ACA because of their curved course. Typical spectra recorded from the PCA and ACA are shown in **Figures 26.4** and **26.5**. **Table 26.2** shows normal values (mean ± standard deviation) for the flow velocities in circle of Willis arteries, scanning angles, and associated measurement errors [2.3].

Normal values for circle of Willis arteries				
Criteria	MCA	ACA	PCA	BA
PSV [cm/s]	107 ± 14	98 ± 15	75 ± 17	58 ± 14
Scan angle [°]	33 ± 15	35 ± 17	45 ± 18	15 ± 14
Error [%]	15	18	30	3

Table 26.2

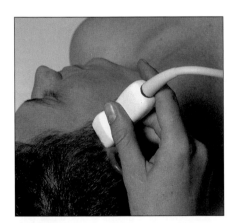

Fig. 26.1a

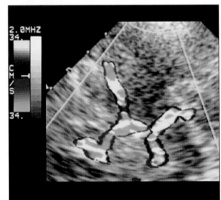

Fig. 26.1b

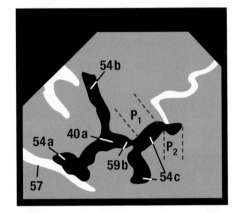

Fig. 26.1c

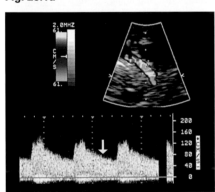

Fig. 26.3

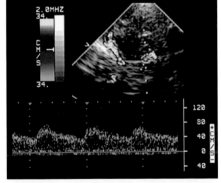

Fig. 26.4

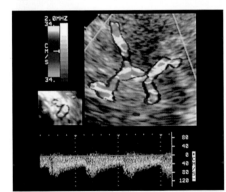

Fig. 26.5

Transnuchal examination of the basilar artery

Transnuchal scanning can be performed in the sitting position with the patient's head flexed forward **(Fig. 25.5a)** or with the patient supine and the head turned to the side. This can demonstrate both V_4 segments **(55)** at their junction with the basilar artery **(56)**. **Figure 26.6a+b** shows a typical duplex display, which here includes a portion of the right posterior inferior cerebellar artery (PICA, **55a**).

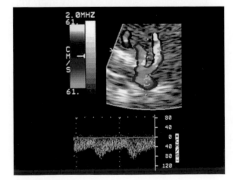

Fig. 26.6a

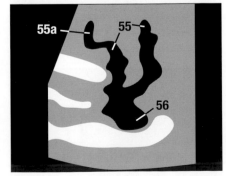

Fig. 26.6b

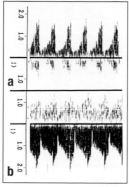

Fig. 27.1

Findings in intracranial vascular disease

In our discussion of extracranial vascular lesions, we noted the importance of intact collateral pathways for assessing preoperative risk and the risk of stroke (see p.20). In patients with high-grade internal carotid stenosis or unilateral internal carotid occlusion, it is also important to determine whether there is retrograde collateral flow through the ophthalmic artery from the ECA territory **(Fig. 27.1b)** as opposed to zero flow or normal flow **(Fig. 27.1a)**. The pattern of intracranial collateralization can be appreciated by comparing the Doppler spectra from specific arteries. **Figure 27.2**, obtained from a patient with an occluded right ICA, shows a decreased PSV (↘) and increased diastolic flow level (⇓) in the ipsilateral MCA **(a)** compared with the left MCA **(b)**. The right MCA is perfused by crossover flow from the anterior communicating artery **(c)** with retrograde flow in the right A_1 segment **(d)**.

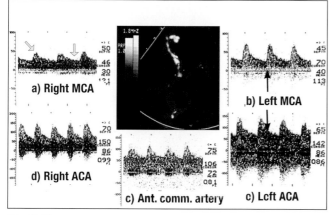

Fig. 27.2

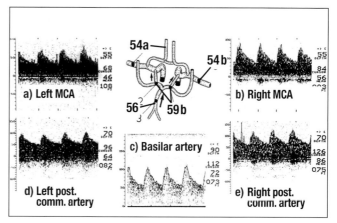

Fig. 27.3

In the case of a bilateral internal carotid occlusion **(Fig. 27.3)**, collateral flow is generally derived from the posterior circulation with an intact circle of Willis or through ophthalmic collaterals **(Fig. 27.1b)**. In the case illustrated, increased flow is detected in the basilar artery **(Fig. 27.3c)**, both posterior communicating arteries **(d, e)**, and both middle cerebral arteries **(a, b)**. This reflects a compensatory flow increase that should not be mistaken for flow acceleration due to stenosis. To avoid misinterpretation, it is always prudent to sample all the major circle of Willis arteries that are accessible to Doppler examination.

Flow acceleration can have causes other than stenosis. Anemia, for example, can induce a functional flow acceleration (↖) in the ICA **(Fig. 27.4)**, as shown here for a patient with a hemoglobin of just 6.2 g/dl. Aneurysms can also cause flow acceleration and can be detected with CDS when larger than 5-10 mm and located at an accessible site. **Figure 27.5** shows an approximately 1-cm-large aneurysm **(8)** located in the distal M_1 segment of the right middle cerebral artery **(54b)**.

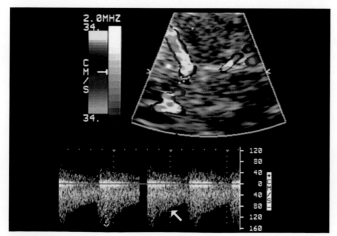

Fig. 27.4

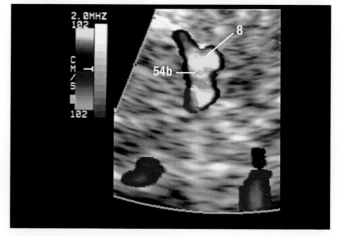

Fig. 27.5

Critical evaluation

With their superficial location and the ability to achieve good image resolution at high frequencies, the carotid arteries are ideal for noninvasive color duplex evaluation. To a degree, this also applies to the vertebral arteries. The origin of the left vertebral artery, often located at a relatively low site, can be particularly difficult to evaluate with CDS. A similar problem exists in the approximately 4% of cases where the vertebral artery springs directly from the aortic arch. An alternative noninvasive technique for excluding a vertebral or carotid artery dissection is MR angiography (MRA), which can be performed using the time-of-flight method (TOF MRA) or contrast administration. **Figure 28.1** demonstrates an occlusion of the left ICA with associated collateral channels. It is important to evaluate the individual axial partitions and not just the 3-D reconstructions to reliably exclude an intimal flap.

Another, more invasive option is DSA **(Fig. 28.2)**, the main advantages of which are its ability to detect slow residual flow in very tight stenoses and define the lumina of small intracranial vessels. This case illustrates a small aneurysm (↖). DSA can also demonstrate collaterals and venous drainage for exclusion of dural sinus thrombosis.

In up to 15% of cases, cranial penetration by Doppler ultrasound is so severely hampered (e.g., by a thick calvarium) that contrast agents should be used. Compare the apparent cutoff of the MCA (✐) without contrast administration in **Figure 28.3a** with the improved signal-to-noise ratio following the administration of Levovist in **Figure 28.3b**. The postcontrast scan shows that the lesion is not an occlusion but a high-grade MCA stenosis with associated flow acceleration (⇐).

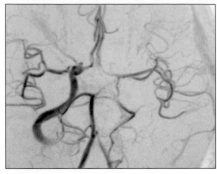

Fig. 28.1

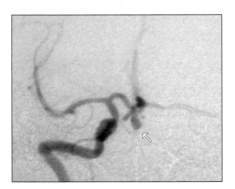

Fig. 28.2

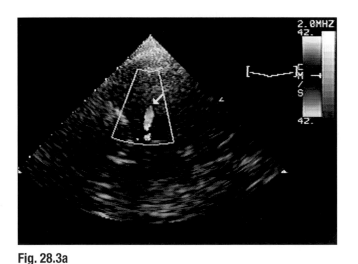

Fig. 28.3a

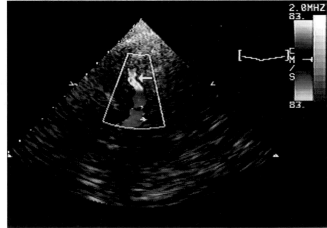

Fig. 28.3b

Quiz – Take the following quiz to test your knowledge:

1. Name three collateral pathways that may be evoked by an internal carotid stenosis or vertebral artery stenosis. Check your answers on p.18.

2. Draw from memory the normal spectral waveforms of the CCA, ICA, and ECA. Compare your drawings with **Figures 20.4 - 20.6**.

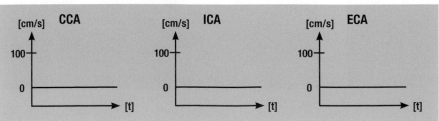

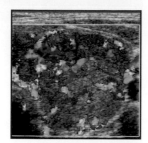

Andreas Saleh

Introduction

The cervical lymph nodes are so superficial that they can be imaged with a high-frequency (5-10 MHz) linear transducer. Their accessibility to detailed imaging significantly expands the spectrum of analytic criteria (see p. 30) compared with the ultrasound examination of abdominal lymph nodes. The presence of lymph node metastases is a critical prognostic factor in patients with head and neck tumors, and the nodal stage significantly influences therapeutic decision making. Thoracic tumors can also metastasize to cervical lymph nodes and often affect staging. The staging of malignant lymphoma encompasses all nodal stations in the body including the cervical nodes.

Thyroid diseases are very common in geographic regions with endemic iodine deficiency. Ultrasonography is the initial imaging study performed in patients with suspected thyroid disease. With endemic diffuse goiter, the thyroid gland is enlarged but shows otherwise normal echogenicity and color duplex features. In patients with a new occurrence of Graves' disease, hyperthyroidism is present as the dominant clinical symptom. Often the diffuse low echogenicity of the thyroid is so typical that the

B-mode image itself will suggest the correct diagnosis. CDS almost always shows a degree of hypervascularity that is sufficient to confirm Graves' disease. The sonographic appearance of thyroiditis is less specific. Areas of inflammatory infiltration are hypoechoic and show central or peripheral hypervascularity, but these changes are less pronounced than in Graves' disease. Every focal lesion of the thyroid should be investigated as a possible autonomous adenoma or thyroid malignancy. At present, CDS does not provide reliable criteria for either the functional evaluation or the benign-malignant differentiation of a thyroid nodule.

Anatomy

The search for cervical lymph nodes is aided by subdividing the neck into regions that can be systematically surveyed with ultrasound **(Fig. 29.1)**. The submental trigone extends along the cervical midline from the hyoid bone **(21d)** to the chin and is bounded laterally by the anterior bellies of the digastric muscles **(47a)**. Adjacent to this trigone is the submandibular trigone, which is bounded by the anterior belly **(47a)** and posterior belly **(47b)** of the digastric and by the mandible. The lymph nodes in both regions are called level I nodes in the surgical terminology of neck dissection. Next to be examined are the lymph nodes along the internal jugular vein **(41a)**, which are designated as levels II-IV in the craniocaudal direction. The lateral cervical triangle is bounded by the posterior border of the sternocleidomastoid muscle **(44)**, the anterior border of the trapezius muscle, and by the clavicle **(21c)** (level V) and includes the supraclavicular fossa. The anterior cervical triangle extends from the hyoid bone **(21d)** to the infraclavicular fossa and is bounded laterally by the sternocleidomastoid muscle **(44)** (level VI). Visualization of the nuchal and mastoid lymph nodes completes the survey protocol.

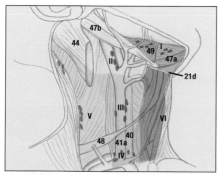

Fig. 29.1

Examination technique

As lymph nodes are encountered during the examination, they are individually evaluated. This is done by rotating the transducer to demonstrate the lymph node in its longest axis **(Fig. 30.1)**. This maximum longitudinal diameter is bisected by the perpendicular transverse diameter. The resulting M/T ratio (ratio of longest diameter to transverse diameter) characterizes the shape of the lymph node. A node with an M/T ratio < 2 has an approximately spherical shape, raising suspicion of metastatic involvement. This criterion is not reliable for lymph nodes smaller than 1 cm, because the measurement error is too large. Additionally, lymph node metastases smaller than 1 cm or larger than 4 cm are frequently nonspherical. Lymph nodes larger than 4 cm are suspicious by their maximum diameter alone. Thus, the M/T ratio is most useful for lymph nodes with a maximum diameter of 1-2 cm, in which a broad overlap exists between benign and malignant

B-mode criteria for lymph node evaluation
Size
Shape (M/T ratio)
Central hilar echo
Echogenicity
Margins

Table 30.1

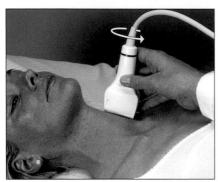

Fig. 30.1a

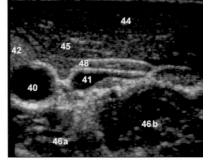

Fig. 30.1b

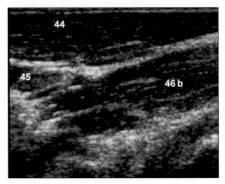

Fig. 30.1c

nodes [3.5]. Normal lymph nodes and nodes affected with nonspecific lymphadenitis display a hypoechoic cortex **(50b)** with a bright central hilar echo **(50a) (Fig. 30.5)**. With nodal metastases and malignant lymphoma, the hilar echo is absent in 50-80% of cases. Malignant lymphoma is usually associated with a very hypoechoic cortex, which may even appear pseudocystic. Nodal metastases often exhibit a complex echo structure due to regressive changes. Lymph nodes are almost always sharply marginated, but metastases may occasionally have ill-defined margins.

Color duplex criteria for lymph node evaluation
Degree of vascularity
Vascular distribution pattern
Pulsatility of intranodal blood flow

Table 30.2

For the color duplex evaluation of a lymph node, visualize the intranodal vessels in the color Doppler mode. Evaluate both the degree and pattern of the vascularity. Then place the sample volume in the largest vessels **(51a)** and record a Doppler frequency spectrum **(Fig. 30.4)**. Angle correction is unnecessary, because only the pulsatility parameters RI and PI are of interest. Lymph-node metastases from squamous-cell carcinoma (SCC) have a higher resistance index than benign lymph nodes. With RI > 0.8 and PI > 1.6, lymph node metastasis can be diagnosed with a sensitivity of approximately 55% and a specificity of approximately 95% [3.3]. The higher resistance in lymph node metastases results from the obstruction of peripheral vascular channels by invading tumor cells. Both malignant lymphoma and lymphadenitis are characterized by a low resistance index (RI < 0.8).

Features of normal lymph nodes
Size < 1.5 cm
Oblong shape (M/T ratio > 2)
Bright hilar echo
Sharp margins
No detectable vascularity in color-flow image

Table 30.3

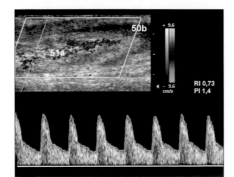

Fig. 30.4

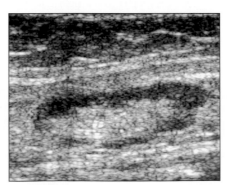

Fig. 30.5a

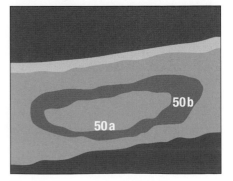

Fig. 30.5b

Figure 31.1a shows a 3.5cm cervical lymph node in Hodgkin disease. The node is so sonolucent that it causes marked posterior acoustic enhancement **(20)**. A hilar echo is not seen. **Figure 31.1b** shows a 3-D reconstruction of the intranodal blood vessels. The node is markedly hypervascular, with vessels extending to the nodal periphery and showing an orderly, arborizing pattern.

Features of malignant lymphoma

Spherical shape (M/T ratio < 2)
Markedly low echogenicity
Frequent absence of hilar echo
Sharp margins
Marked hypervascularity
Arborizing intranodal vascular pattern
Intranodal RI < 0.8

Table 31.1

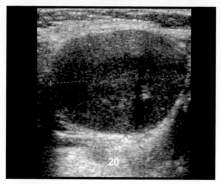

Fig. 31.1a

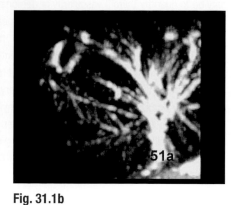

Fig. 31.1b

Figure 31.2 shows a 5.5cm cervical nodal metastasis from SCC. The lesion has ill-defined margins and blends imperceptibly with healthy tissue in the lower right portion of the image (compare with the sharply marginated lymph node in **Fig. 31.1**). The lesion is only moderately vascularized in relation to its size, the vessels radiating from the periphery of the node toward the center. This spoked-wheel pattern of vascularity is always pathologic. A hilar echo **(50a)** is not visible.

Features of lymph node metastasis from squamous cell carcinoma (SCC)

Spherical shape (M/T ratio < 2)
Hypoechoic, regressive change
No hilar echo
Possible ill-defined margins
Scant vascularity
Irregular vascular pattern
Intranodal RI > 0.8

Table 31.2

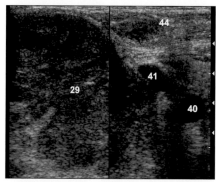

Fig. 31.2a

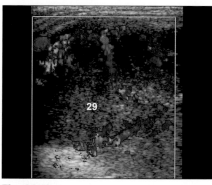

Fig. 31.2b

Figure 31.3 shows a lymph node in acute lymphadenitis. The greater vascularity of acute lymphadenitis is the only feature that distinguishes it from chronic lymphadenitis **(Fig. 31.4)**. A lymph node in chronic lymphadenitis differs from a normal lymph node **(Table 30.3)** only in its size.

Features of acute lymphadenitis

Oblong shape (M/T ratio >> 2)
Cortex slightly hypoechoic
Central hilar echo
Sharp margins
Hypervascularity
Central hilar vessel
Intranodal RI < 0.8

Table 31.3

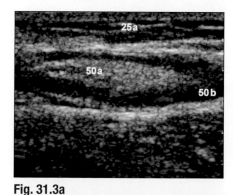

Fig. 31.3a

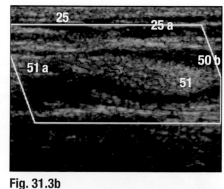

Fig. 31.3b

Features of chronic lymphadenitis

Oblong shape (M/T ratio >> 2)
Cortex slightly hypoechoic
Central hilar echo
Sharp margins
No detectable vascularity

Table 31.4

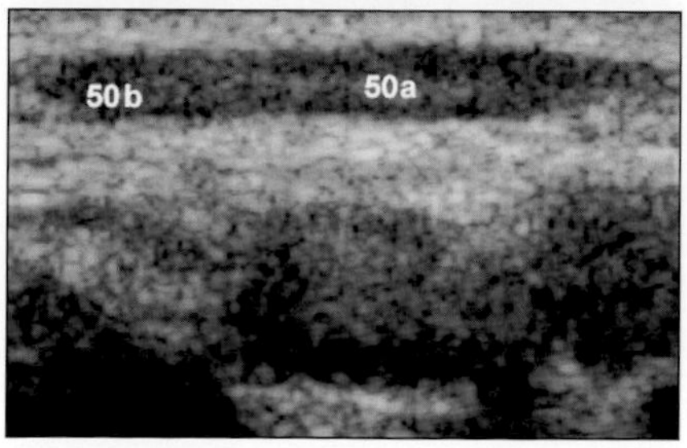

Fig. 31.4a

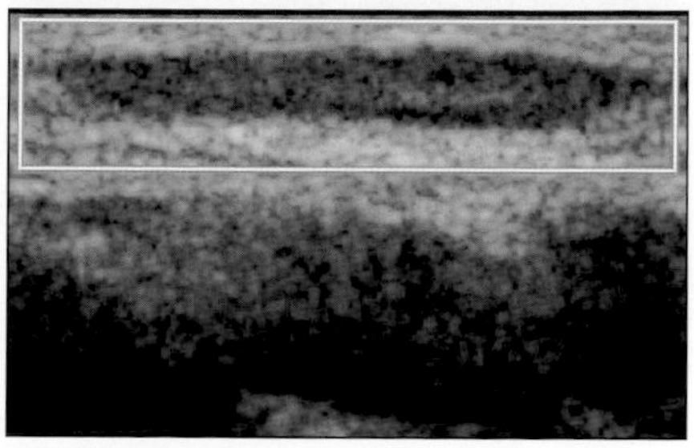

Fig. 31.4b

Doppler examination technique

The vascularity of the thyroid gland **(42)** can be assessed with color flow and pulsed Doppler. Depending on the clinical problem (diffuse or focal thyroid disease), the goal of the examination may be to quantify thyroid vascularity or demonstrate its vascular architecture.

Pulsed Doppler is used to measure peak systolic velocity and volume flow in the thyroid arteries. The inferior thyroid artery **(43b)** makes a bend posterior to the common carotid artery (CCA, **40**). The apex of the bend consistently appears as a vascular cross section (⇡) in a longitudinal scan over the CCA **(Fig. 32.1)**. The transducer can now be slightly rotated to image the descending limb of the inferior thyroid artery, and the Doppler sample volume is positioned within that segment **(Fig. 32.3)**. The superior thyroid artery **(43a)**, located just medial to the CCA at the upper pole of the thyroid gland, is imaged with a slightly modified longitudinal scan **(Fig. 32.4)**. It is easily identified by its opposite flow direction relative to the adjacent CCA. The thyroid vessels normally have a peak systolic velocity of 25 cm/s and a volume flow of 6 ml/min per vessel [3.1].

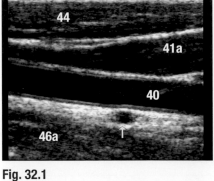

Fig. 32.1

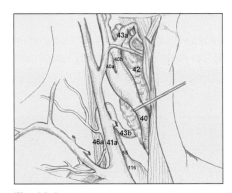

Fig. 32.2

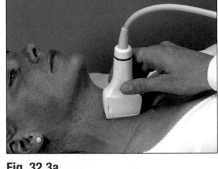

Fig. 32.3a

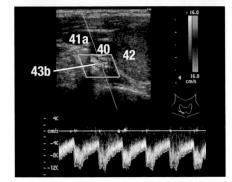

Fig. 32.3b

Diffuse thyroid disease can be evaluated by placing the color box over a representative section of the thyroid gland **(42)**. This permits a semiquantitative assessment of parenchymal blood flow. Standard instrument settings will ensure inter- and intraindividual consistency. This cannot be accomplished if different machines or different settings are used. Every examiner, therefore, should become experienced on a particular machine before trying to assess the degree of increased blood flow. All the images in this chapter were acquired at either a flow-sensitive setting (PRF 1000 Hz, color gain 78%) or an insensitive setting (PRF 2500 Hz, color gain 60%). All the images for a particular category can be compared, therefore. **Figure 32.5** shows normal color duplex findings obtained at the sensitive **(b)** and insensitive settings **(c)**.

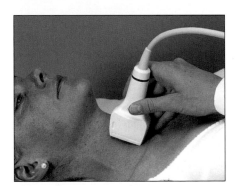

Fig. 32.4a

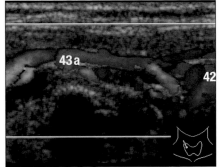

Fig. 32.4b

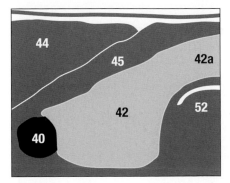

Fig. 32.5a

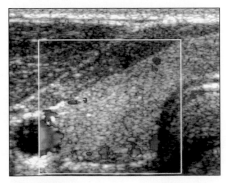

Fig. 32.5b

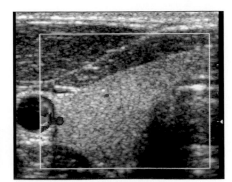

Fig. 32.5c

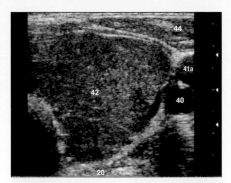

Fig. 33.1a

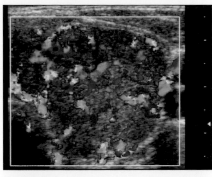

Fig. 33.1b

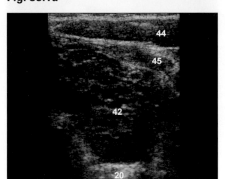

Fig. 33.2a

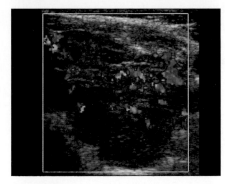

Fig. 33.2b

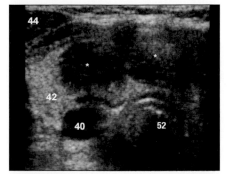

Fig. 33.3a

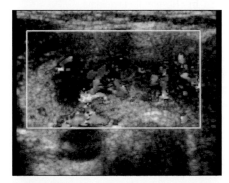

Fig. 33.3b

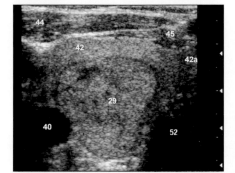

Fig. 33.4a

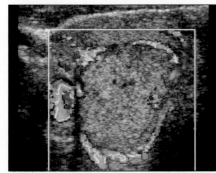

Fig. 33.4b

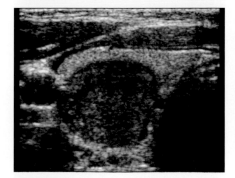

Fig. 33.5a

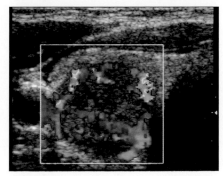

Fig. 33.5b

The diffuse hypervascularity in florid Graves' disease is so pronounced that it may be considered pathognomonic for the disease [3.4]. The peak systolic velocities average more than 100 cm/s, the volume flow more than 150 ml/min. **Figure 33.1** shows the typical B-mode and color-flow features of Graves' disease at the insensitive color setting (see **Fig. 32.5c**). Even when a euthyroid state has been established by medical treatment, the increased blood flow in the thyroid gland initially persists and will decline only with passage of time.

Hashimoto thyroiditis (**Fig. 33.2**) has a similar B-mode appearance. Color flow at the sensitive setting shows a definite increase in blood flow (see **Fig. 32.5b**), but the increase is less pronounced than in florid Graves' disease.

In de Quervain thyroiditis (**Fig. 33.3**), the inflammation usually does not involve the entire thyroid gland but infiltrates the gland in a nonhomogeneous pattern. The sonographic correlate is a disordered pattern of hypoechoic and hypervascular areas (*).

Nodular hyperplasia usually presents with hyperechoic and isoechoic nodules. A hypoechoic rim (halo) is frequently present, but in contrast to focal hepatic lesions it does not imply malignancy. The halo does not always correspond to a ringlike hypervascular pattern as shown in **Fig. 33.4b**. In some cases this pattern may occur in the absence of a B-mode halo. Although most autonomous adenomas (**Fig. 33.4**) show ringlike hypervascularity, this sign is nonspecific and is also seen with nodular hyperplasia and carcinoma.

Most thyroid carcinomas are hypoechoic with peripheral and central hypervascularity (**Fig. 33.5**). To justify a suspicion of malignancy, the sonographic criteria for malignancy must be interpreted in relation to radionuclide findings (cold spot) and clinical parameters.

Critical evaluation

The standard imaging modality for head and neck tumors is CT, which permits simultaneous examination of the primary tumor and regional lymph nodes. In CT, however, nodal size and possible rim enhancement after contrast administration are the only criteria that can be used for benign-malignant differentiation. If nodal sizes are in the "gray area," CT should be supplemented by ultrasound owing to the numerous analytic criteria that are available with that modality.

Ultrasound in malignant lymphoma is an effective modality for the staging of neck disease. One disadvantage is that the results are not as easily documented as in CT. Also, ultrasound cannot evaluate the lymphatic tissue in Waldeyer's ring, which can swell in systemic lymphatic diseases and cause potentially hazardous pharyngeal constriction (**Fig. 34.1**, arrowheads).

CDS cannot provide definitive information on the functional status of thyroid nodules or their benign-malignant differentiation. In this respect it does not compete with fine-needle aspiration biopsy or radionuclide imaging. In diffuse thyroid diseases and especially in Graves' disease, CDS can help to assess the inflammatory activity of the disease and, when combined with laboratory findings, is therefore useful for diagnosis and follow-up.

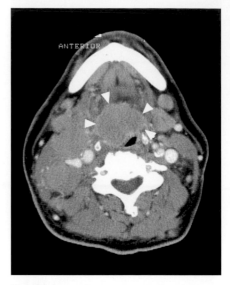

Fig. 34.1

Quiz – Take the following quiz to test your knowledge:

1. Describe the ultrasound features of:
- **a)** a normal lymph node
- **b)** a lymph node involved by malignant lymphoma
- **c)** a lymph node metastasis from SCC
- **d)** acute lymphadenitis
- **e)** chronic lymphadenitis

2. Describe the ultrasound features of:
- **a)** Graves' disease
- **b)** Hashimoto thyroiditis
- **c)** de Quervain thyroiditis
- **d)** nodular hyperplasia

3. In the examination of a woman with clinical manifestations of hyperthyroidism, scanning at the insensitive color-flow setting yields the findings shown below **(Fig. 34.2)**. Describe the findings. What is your diagnosis?

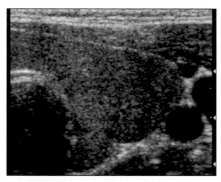

Fig. 34.2a

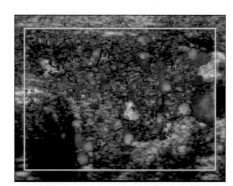

Fig. 34.2b

4. Figure 34.3 shows an inguinal lymph node in a patient with a diabetic foot ulcer. **Figure 34.4** shows cervical lymph nodes in a patient with clinically indeterminate neck masses. Describe both findings, using all the analytic criteria. What are your diagnoses?

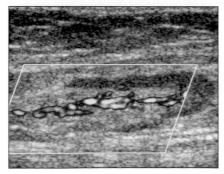

Fig. 34.3

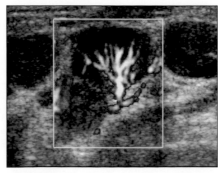

Fig. 34.4

The answers are on pages 31, 33 and at the back of the book.

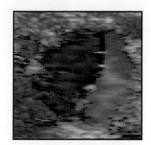

Ghazaleh Tabatabai
Matthias Hofer

Introduction

Flow detection by CDS has expanded the capabilities of abdominal ultrasound. The use of CDS is based on established clinical indications that require a specific examination protocol and quantification of flow, as in the postinterventional follow-up of TIPSS insertions (p. 41). Also, color flow can be activated at any time during the ultrasound examination to determine the vascular nature of indeterminate hypoechoic or anechoic structures.

In abdominal ultrasound, the examiner is confronted with a great variety of clinical problems and vascular territories. The instrument settings should always be carefully adjusted to optimize the display. The known standard planes are frequently varied so that tortuous vessels can be scanned at a favorable Doppler angle.

This chapter deals with the normal ultrasound appearance of abdominal vascular territories as well as pathologic findings based on selected illustrative cases. The diagnosis of parenchymal disease is limited to hepatic lesions because of their unique clinical importance. Our goal is not to cover abdominal CDS completely but to review its key aspects and thus provide an introduction to this complex field.

Sonographic anatomy of the aorta and its branches

The abdominal aorta **(AO, 30)** descends on the left side of the vertebral column from the aortic aperture of the diaphragm to the level of the L4 vertebra, where it bifurcates into the common iliac arteries **(127)**. Its diameter tapers from less than 25 mm at the subdiaphragmatic level to less than 20 mm at the level of the bifurcation [4.1].

The first unpaired visceral branch of the abdominal aorta, the celiac trunk **(71)**, usually arises to the left of the midline **(Fig. 38.2)**. It curves slightly to the right before dividing into the approximately equal-caliber common hepatic artery **(CHA, 67a)**, the splenic artery **(SA, 71c)**, and the small-caliber left gastric artery **(71a)**. The CHA takes a meandering course in the hepatoduodenal ligament to the liver, passing in front of the portal vein **(PV, 62)**. The splenic artery, accompanied by the homonymous vein, runs along the posterior border of the pancreas to the hilum of the spleen.

The superior mesenteric artery **(SMA, 72a)** usually arises from the AO about 1 cm distal to the celiac trunk. Its main trunk runs parallel to the AO and can be traced with ultrasound for a considerable distance **(Fig. 36.2)** while the mesenteric vascular arcades are no longer seen.

The inferior mesenteric artery **(IMA, 72b)** arises about 4 cm above the aortic bifurcation **(30d)** and runs a short course to the left of the AO before dividing into its branches **(Fig. 38.4)**. Bühler's anastomosis unites the celiac trunk with the SMA via the pancreaticoduodenal arteries. The SMA and IMA anastomose via the middle and left colic arteries (Riolan's anastomosis).

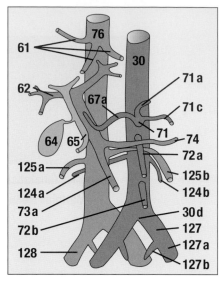

Fig. 36.1

Examination technique

The patient is examined supine with a convex transducer array at an intermediate frequency (usually 3.5 MHz). A roll behind the knee increases patient comfort and improves scanning conditions by relaxing the abdominal wall. The entire AO is imaged first in longitudinal and transverse B-mode sections and then with color flow. Finally, Doppler spectra are acquired for the quantification of stenoses. A typical upper abdominal longitudinal scan in **Figure 36.2a** demonstrates the proximal AO **(30)**, the origin of the celiac trunk **(71)**, and the SMA **(72a)**.

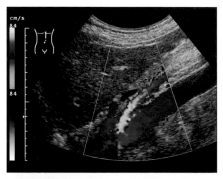

Fig. 36.2a

Normal findings

The flow pattern in the AO is not uniform. At the suprarenal level **(Fig. 36.3a)** the systolic peak (⟹) is followed by constant forward flow in diastole (⇧). But a scan at the infrarenal level **(Fig. 36.3b)** normally shows early diastolic flow reversal (↖) like that in peripheral arteries. This should not be mistaken for pathologic flow reversal or aliasing.

Flow velocities in the AO are approximately 50 cm/s slower than in peripheral arteries because of the large aortic caliber. The velocities and reverse flow component are subject to large interindividual variations [4.1].

Color-flow imaging of the infrarenal aorta is often unsuccessful in the upper abdominal longitudinal scan (↘ , **Fig. 36.3a**), because the angle between the sound path (↓) and flow direction (↗) is unfavorable (90°) when a convex array is used, and transducer angulation can do little to improve the situation. Shifting the transducer caudad gives

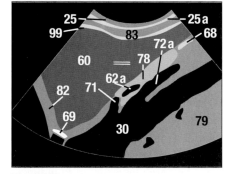

Fig. 36.2b

a more favorable Doppler angle **(Fig. 36.3b)**, but the gas-filled transverse colon often interferes with scanning at the midabdominal level. The most common aortic lesion is atherosclerosis. CDS can demonstrate the hemodynamics of associated changes such as stenosis, occlusion, and aneurysms.

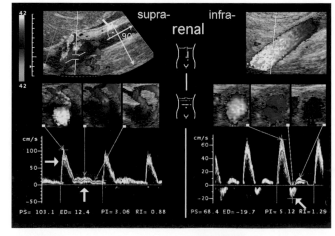

Fig. 36.3a **Fig. 36.3b**

Criteria for aortic dilatation (bold type: risk of rupture)

1. Flow laminar or **turbulent**

2. Max. AO diameter: < 2.5 cm
   Indication for surgery: **> 5 cm, progression of > 0.5 cm/year**

3. Width and location of perfused, thrombosed or false lumen:
   eccentric location

4. Involvement of renal, visceral, or iliac arteries?
   (surgical strategy and implant selection)

5. Peripheral aneurysmosis? (see Chap. 8)

6. Spectra in true and false lumen?
   (impending ischemia, indication for surgery)

Table 36.4

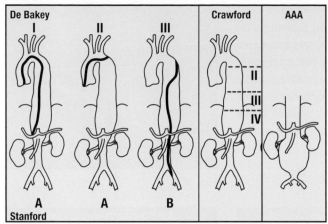

Fig. 37.1a b c

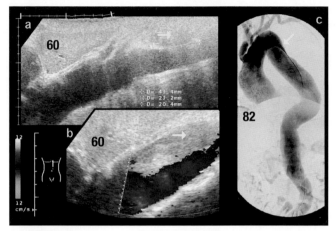

Fig. 37.2a–2c

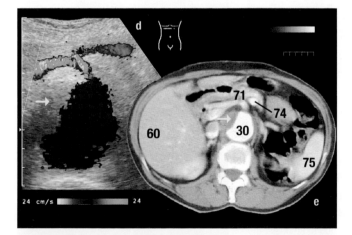

Fig. 37.2d, 2e

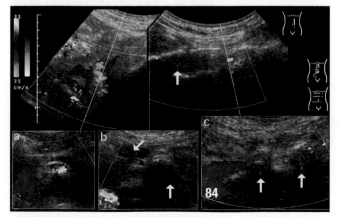

Fig. 37.4

Aneurysms

An abdominal aortic aneurysm (AAA) is often clinically silent. Further enlargement and peripheral emboli lead to nonspecific symptoms such as backache or abdominal pain. If an AAA is detected incidentally at ultrasound or is investigated electively, the criteria listed in **Table 36.4** are documented to provide a baseline for monitoring growth tendency and rupture risk and assessing the need for surgical treatment.

Classification

An isolated AAA is common and is usually located at the infrarenal level. There may be concomitant involvement of the iliac circulation. The spatial extent of the less common thoracoabdominal aneurysm forms the basis for Crawford's four-stage classification **(Fig. 37.1b)**. A type I aneurysm (not shown) does not involve the infrarenal aorta. Stages II through IV define the level (---) of thoracic involvement by an aneurysm with infrarenal extension.

Figure 37.2 shows the appearance of a thoracoabdominal aneurysm with partial marginal thrombosis in DSA **(c)**, CT **(e)**, SieScape **(a)**, and in longitudinal **(b)** and transverse **(d)** color-flow images. The AO aneurysm and marginal thrombosis (⟹) are clearly defined with ultrasound. Information on the extent of thoracic involvement and spatial relationships for preoperative planning is furnished by Doppler spectra **(c**, ✓ = catheter) and CT **(e)**.

With a dissecting aneurysm **(Fig. 37.4)**, blood dissects between the intima and media through a rent in the vessel wall. An intimal flap (↗) separates the true and false lumina and floats in the blood stream (↗ Doppler signal). The extent of the aneurysm can be defined by CT or DSA using the Stanford or DeBakey classification **(Fig. 37.1a)**. CDS can furnish additional information on the involvement of splanchnic and pelvic arteries and can also be used for close-interval follow-up.

Leriche syndrome

Leriche syndrome refers to an occlusion of the AO that involves the iliac bifurcation **(Fig. 37.3)**. Longitudinal and transverse scans **(a)** at the level of the SMA origin still demonstrate flow. Farther distally, however, an absence of flow signals (⇑) is found in transverse scans at the level of the mesenteric root (✓ **b**) and caudal to the bifurcation **(c**, with reference marks). Note that local color voids may result from an unfavorable scanning angle or from anterior shadowing plaques. Faulty instrument settings can lead to false-positive findings. Collateralization to the leg through epigastric vessels is shown in **Figure 78.5** (Chapter 7).

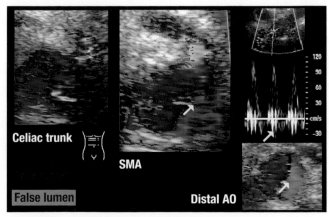

Fig. 37.5

Examination of the splanchnic arteries

The splanchnic arteries should be examined in the fasting state (see below). Scanning at full expiration rather than full inspiration often provides good visualization. Pathologic findings are documented with spectral traces, and the measured flow velocities are interpreted in relation to aortic flow. Direct color-flow imaging will occasionally make it easier to locate small vessels. But color flow also delays real-time visualization (do you know why? See the introductory chapter), and moving the transducer around to search for vessels can increase color artifacts. **Figure 38.2a** illustrates the search for the correct transverse planes, the location of which is marked with lines in the upper abdominal longitudinal scan **(Fig. 38.1)**.

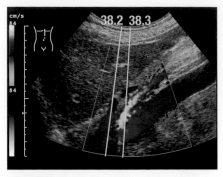

Fig. 38.1

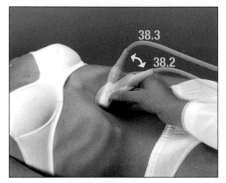

Fig. 38.2a

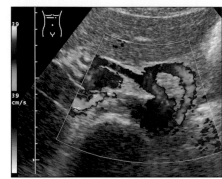

Fig. 38.2b

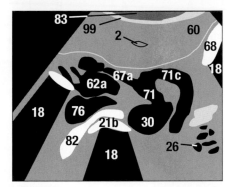

Fig. 38.2c

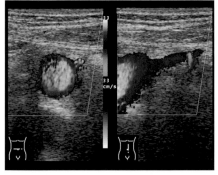

Fig. 38.4

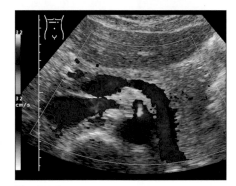

Fig. 38.3a

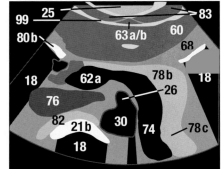

Fig. 38.3b

Normal findings

The splanchnic arteries show a combination of blue- and red-encoded segments, depending on whether flow is directed toward or away from the transducer (see **71c**, **Fig. 38.2b**). Apparent velocity increases may be found at sites such as the SMA origin, where blood is flowing directly toward the transducer, resulting in brighter colors (**26**, **Figs. 38.1** and **38.3**) or even aliasing (⇓ **Fig. 38.5**). As the SMA origin is also a common site of flow acceleration due to stenosis, the velocity spectrum should be analyzed carefully to differentiate artifacts from true stenosis (see **Table 39.3**).

A 5-MHz transducer is advantageous in thin patients. The higher resolution and the capacity for beam steering with linear transducers make it easier to visualize structures such as the IMA origin **(Fig. 38.4)** [4.2].

Flow in the splanchnic arteries varies with food intake and respirations. Postprandial examination shows a significant increase in peak systolic velocity (PSV) and end-diastolic flow (ED), although these effects are less pronounced in the celiac trunk than in the SMA, for example [4.3]. While the SMA spectrum often shows a definite triphasic pattern in the fasting state **(Fig. 38.5a)**, it becomes biphasic following a meal **(Fig. 38.5b)**. A lack of spectral change after the administration of a test meal has diagnostic implications.

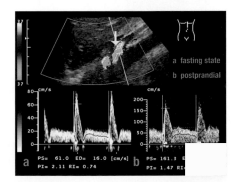

Fig. 38.5a   **Fig. 38.5b**

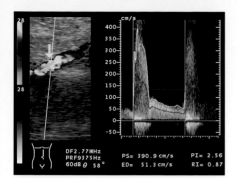

Fig. 39.1

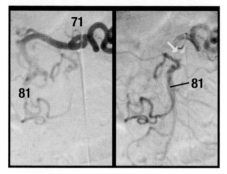

Fig. 39.2

Criteria for stenosis of the SMA and celiac trunk (measured in the fasting state)		
PSV	Celiac trunk	> 200 cm/s
	SMA	> 270 cm/s
PDV	Celiac trunk	> 100 cm/s
	SMA	> 70 cm/s
PSV-ratio	$\dfrac{\text{PSV SMA}}{\text{PSV AO}}$	> 3.5

Table 39.3

Intestinal ischemia

Chronic bowel ischemia can remain asymptomatic for years due to collateral circulation. But if plaque thrombosis or embolization occurs, acute ischemia can develop. Because of its location, the SMA is the most commonly affected mesenteric vessel.

The differential diagnosis includes nonocclusive bowel ischemia caused by postoperative or pharmacologically induced vasospasm, which is demonstrable by DSA. Color duplex cannot exclude acute mesenteric occlusion, because often it can demonstrate only the origins of the splanchnic arteries, especially if there is associated meteorism and pain. If CDS of the SMA trunk shows an abrupt cutoff of color flow with no detectable spectral trace, SMA occlusion should be diagnosed if it is consistent with clinical and laboratory findings (elevated serum lactic acid).

Collaterals are frequently detected, but DSA is necessary for complete mapping of the collateral circulation (**Fig.39.2**). The occluded SMA ( ) is opacified by retrograde flow through Bühler's anastomosis **(81)**.

CDS can contribute to the investigation of chronic intestinal ischemia. The proximal SMA is a site of predilection for stenosis and is easily examined with color duplex in most patients. The systolic and diastolic flow velocities are important parameters for the quantification of stenosis (see **Table 39.3**). **Figure 39.1** shows a high-grade SMA stenosis with aliasing ( ), pronounced intrastenotic flow acceleration up to 400 cm/s.

The measured peak velocities are expressed in relation to the PSV in the AO. This ratio corrects for any generalized increase in blood flow velocity (e.g., in hyperthyroid patients). Inflammatory bowel disease, tumors (see p. 42), and portal vein thrombosis (see p. 40) also lead to hyperemia in the splanchnic arteries [4.15]. Besides the PSV, the peak diastolic velocity (PDV) is a useful indicator of stenosis. There are still problems in quantifying the degree of stenosis with CDS, however [4.3, 4.4]. Normal values and criteria for stenoses are reviewed in Chapter 1 and **Table 39.3**.

Arcuate ligament compression syndrome

Patients with this syndrome (predominantly seen in thin young women) often present with nonspecific abdominal complaints that usually resolve spontaneously. The problem is caused by proximal constriction of the celiac trunk ( ) by pressure from the diaphragm crus **(82)** in full expiration [4.5]. Note the dependence of flow on the respiratory cycle in **Figure 39.4a**. **Figure 39.4c** shows DSA with ligament compression syndrom ( ) of celiac trunk.

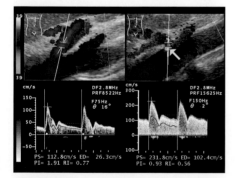

Fig. 39.4a

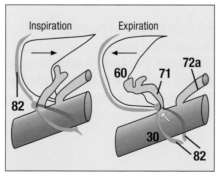

Fig. 39.4b

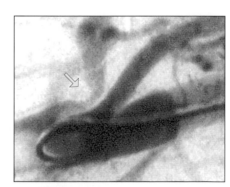

Fig. 39.4c

Aneurysms

Aneurysms of the splanchnic arteries are rare and are usually detected incidentally. The splenic artery and hepatic artery are most commonly affected. False aneurysms (see Chapter 7) can develop in these vessels due to tumor erosion, inflammation, and other causes (see **Fig. 47.5a**).

Vascular prostheses

Vascular prostheses have an echogenic border (**Fig. 39.5**), shown here for a prosthetic graft interposed for celiac trunk occlusion. CDS is a useful noninvasive follow-up study for detecting postoperative complications such as suture aneurysm, anastomotic leak, and occlusion.

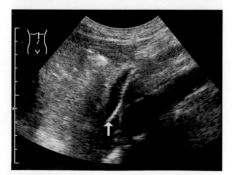

Fig. 39.5

IVC and hepatic veins

Sonographic anatomy

The inferior vena cava **(IVC, 76)** ascends to the right of the spinal column, passing through the diaphragm **(82)** and terminating in the right atrium **(33a)**. Major tributaries that can be imaged with CDS include the iliac veins, the renal veins, and the three hepatic veins **(61)**, which enter the IVC just below the diaphragm **(Fig. 40.1)**. More than three hepatic veins may occur, and the caudate lobe **(60a)** is often drained by a separate vein.

Examination technique

Duplex examination of the IVC usually includes the iliac, renal, and hepatic veins. Once orientation has been established in the B-mode image, the IVC is examined with color flow in two planes along its course. If abnormalities are found, Doppler spectra are recorded for quantitative evaluation.

Normal findings

Flow in the IVC and hepatic veins **(Fig. 40.3a)** shows definite cardiac modulation. Movement of the cardiac valve plane toward the apex in systole creates a strong suction within the atria, inducing rapid flow toward the heart (↗). As the right atrium fills at the start of diastole, venous inflow diminishes (⬇ **Fig. 40.3a**), or a brief period of reverse flow (↙) may even occur **(Fig. 40.3b)**. When the AV valves have opened, blood flows into the ventricles, and the atrium can again receive venous inflow (↖). The atrium contracts at the end of diastole. As there are no valves between the terminating veins and atrium, this contraction of the atrium causes transient flow away from the heart (↘). Closure of the AV valves at end-diastole occasionally produces a small notch (⬅).

Right heart failure can lead to an altered spectral waveform **(Fig. 40.3c)** in which there is a decrease of flow toward the heart. Tricuspid insufficiency (see Chapter 9) leads to pathologic flow reversal in the IVC during systole. Flat, bandlike spectra may be recorded from the hepatic veins in patients with advanced hepatic cirrhosis [4.6].

IVC thrombosis is manifested in the B-mode image by non-compressibility, loss of pulsatility, and hypoechoic dilatation, which appears slightly more echogenic than echo-free lumina. Color flow demonstrates a color void (⬇) in the affected segment **(Fig. 40.4a)**, caused in this example by the extension of thrombosis from the left common iliac vein (CIV) (⬅) **(Fig. 40.4b)**. The right CIV is responsible for the crescent-shaped residual flow (⬆) in the IVC. **Fig. 40.4c** shows complete occlusion **(4)** of IVC resulting from ascending thrombosis.

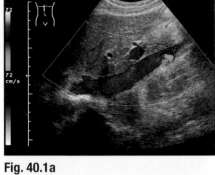

Fig. 40.1a

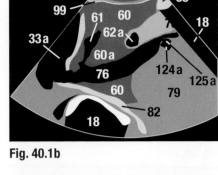

Fig. 40.1b

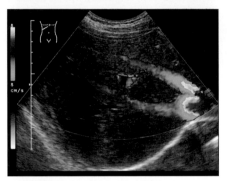

Fig. 40.2a

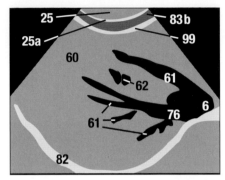

Fig. 40.2b

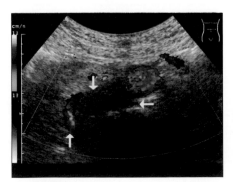

Fig. 40.3a

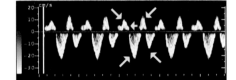

Fig. 40.3b

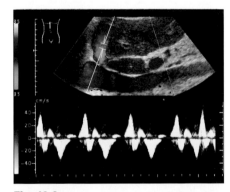

Fig. 40.3c

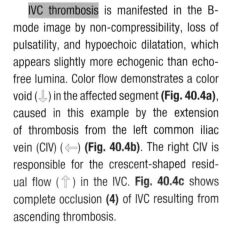

Fig. 40.4a

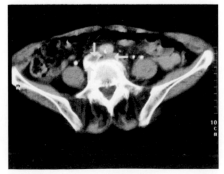

Fig. 40.4b

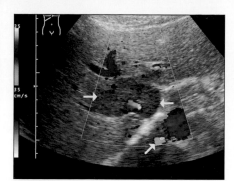

Fig. 41.1a

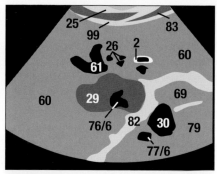

Fig. 41.1b

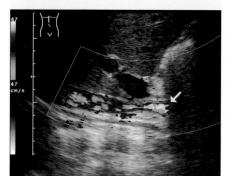

Fig. 41.2a

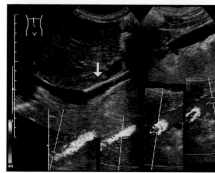

Fig. 41.2b

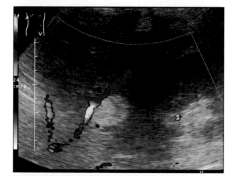

Fig. 41.3a

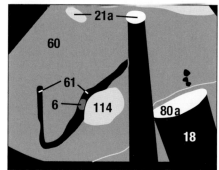

Fig. 41.3b

Vena cava filters can reduce the danger of embolization from the pelvic and lower extremity veins, but complications are frequent. Metal filters placed by transluminal insertion may become dislodged or may thrombose and become a source of emboli [4.7]. CDS can be used in follow-up to determine filter patency.

Luminal narrowing of the IVC may have causes other than thrombosis, including postoperative complications, stenosis, intra-luminal tumor extension (see Chapter 5), and extrinsic compression by tumor. In **Figure 41.1**, the IVC **(76)** is encased (⟹ ⟸) by hepatic metastases **(29)**. This can lead to symptoms of IVC obstruction, here associated with a compensatory flow increase (↗) in the azygos vein **(77)**. One therapeutic option for stenosis is stent insertion (⇓) to improve venous return to the heart **(Fig. 41.2b)**. The preinterventional stenosis (✍) is shown in **Figure 41.2a**.

Hepatic vein thrombosis may affect individual small hepatic veins (veno-occlusive disease, VOD) or the main venous trunks (Budd-Chiari syndrome), with occasional involvement of the IVC. If the thrombosis affects only individual veins or venous segments, an absence of flow on CDS may be accompanied by intersegmental collateralization with a bandlike Doppler spectrum.

Intrahepatic mass lesions such as angioma **(114)** can displace and narrow the hepatic veins on reaching sufficient size **(Fig. 41.3a)**.

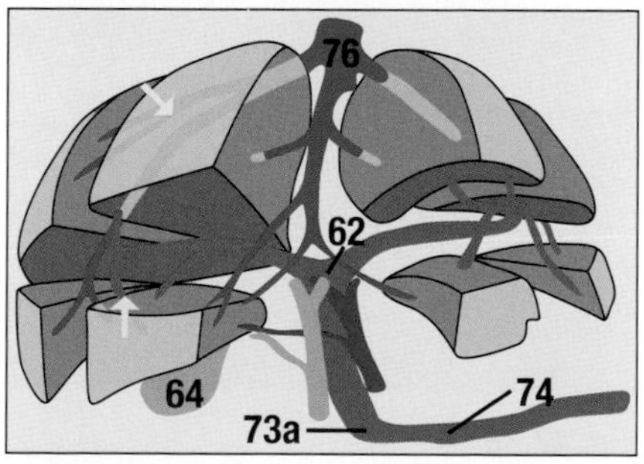

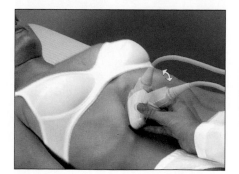

Fig. 41.4a

Portal venous system - sonographic anatomy

The splenic vein **(74)** runs from the hilum of the spleen along the posterior border of the pancreas, accompanied by the homonymous artery. At the confluence, it unites with the superior mesenteric vein (SMV, **73a**) to form the portal vein (PV, **62**) **(Figs. 41.4a, 36.1)**. The intrahepatic branching patterns of the PV (⬆) and hepatic veins (⬂) determine the segmental anatomy of the liver [4.8]. The anatomic diagram **(Fig. 41.4a)** shows the liver from the anterior aspect. The curved arrow ⟳ in **Figure 41.4c** represents the cranial (I) to caudal (II) image position, caused by transducer sweep (⬎) used in **Figure 41.4b** to locate the consecutive planes in the subcostal oblique scan. Coronal MR angiography provides an alternative technique for visualizing the portal venous system **(Fig. 41.4d)**.

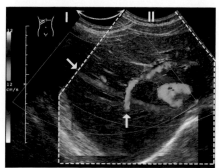

Fig. 41.4b

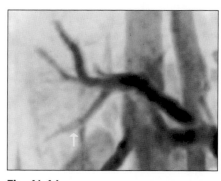

Fig. 41.4c

Fig. 41.4d

Examination technique

The extrahepatic portions of the PV **(62)** are visualized with an extended intercostal scan **(Fig. 42.1)**. If this is unsuccessful due to overlying bowel gas or an unfavorable Doppler angle, the extrahepatic PV can be scanned from a right anterior intercostal approach **(Fig. 42.2)** with the right arm elevated above the head to enlarge the intercostal spaces. Often the periportal main trunk (✎) is visualized only on this plane owing to the favorable acoustic window provided by the liver. The course of the intrahepatic branches is such that they are best visualized with a subcostal oblique scan (see **Fig. 41.4b**). Following the B-mode and color-flow examination, Doppler spectra are recorded to quantify periportal flow in the PV.

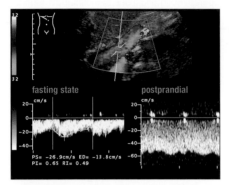

Fig. 42.1a

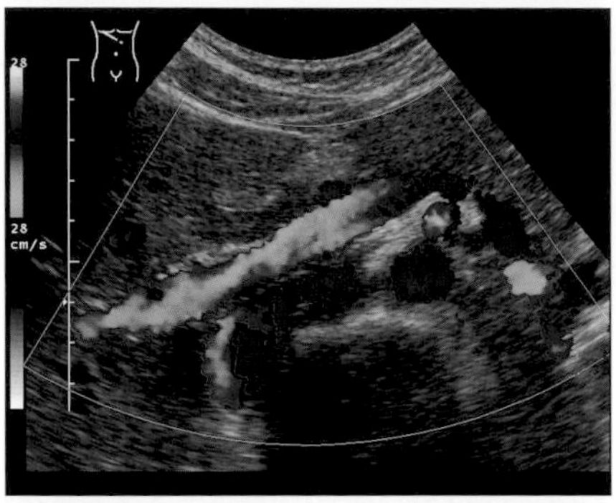

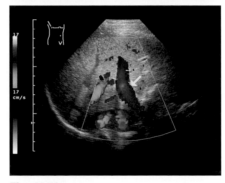

Fig. 42.1b

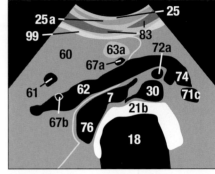

Fig. 42.1c

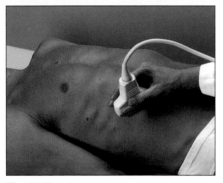

Fig. 42.2a

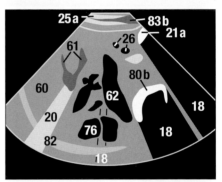

Fig. 42.2b

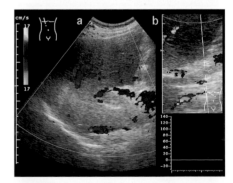

Fig. 42.2c

Normal findings

Color-flow imaging of the PV demonstrates continuous flow toward the liver, which yields a monophasic, bandlike Doppler spectrum. The flow may be modulated by body position and respiration. In particular, flow velocity in the PV is markedly decreased in the sitting position and at full inspiration [4.9]. The peak velocities in **Figure 42.1a** illustrate the effects of fasting and eating on portal venous flow. The flow increases by a factor of at least 1.5 following a meal.

Portal hypertension

Color flow in portal hypertension demonstrates decreased flow or even marked changes such as flow away from the liver in the PV or splenic vein, and it aids in the visualization of collateral pathways **(Table 43.1)**.

Thrombosis **(4)** of the portal vein **(62, Fig. 42.3)** leads to increased resistance in the PV circulation. It may result from cirrhosis, tumor invasion, hypercoagulability, or inflammation. Flow in the proper hepatic artery (PHA, **67b**) increases to compensate for the deficient oxygen supply caused by the failure of portal perfusion. Cavernous transformation may occur along the thrombosed PV, leading to a restoration of hepatopetal flow.

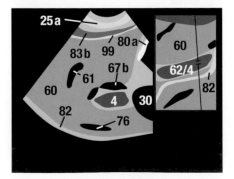

Fig. 42.3a

Fig. 42.3b

Figures 43.3a–c demonstrate collateral channels in portal vein thrombosis. The tortuous venous channels (⬉) pass from the hilum of the spleen along the lesser curvature of the stomach to the esophagus (⬈). Corresponding CT findings are shown in **Figure 43.3b**. A spontaneous splenorenal shunt (⟹ **Fig. 43.2**) may additionally or alternatively develop from small existing veins, or tortuous venous collaterals may form along the obliterated umbilical vein (Cruveilhier-Baumgarten syndrome), with extension to the paraumbilical veins (caput medusae).

Checklist: portal hypertension
Suggestive signs in CDS:
Flow velocity decreased to < 10 cm/s
Thrombosis
Cavernous transformation of the PV
Definite signs in CDS:
Portocaval anastomoses
Flow away from the liver

Table 43.1

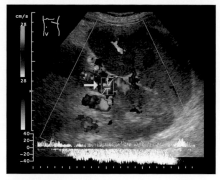

Fig. 43.2a

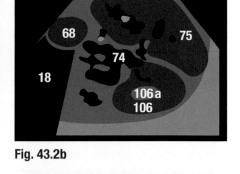

Fig. 43.2b

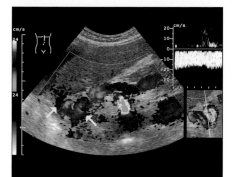

Fig. 43.3a

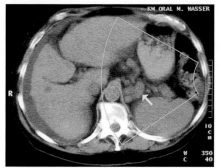

Fig. 43.3b

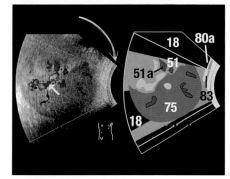

Fig. 43.3c

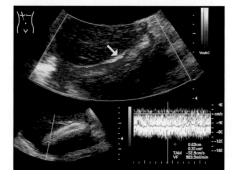

Fig. 43.4

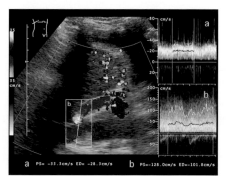

Fig. 43.5

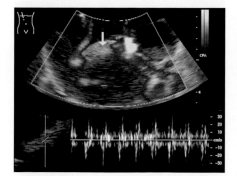

Fig. 43.6

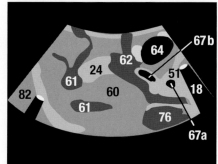

Fig. 43.6a

TIPSS

The insertion of a transjugular intrahepatic portosystemic stent shunt (TIPSS) has become the primary tool for decompression of the portal system. A catheter is advanced through the internal jugular vein into the right hepatic vein and then through the hepatic tissue to the periportal segment of the PV. This communication is held open with a metallic stent. One result of this procedure is a compensatory flow increase in the CHA. Recurring stent stenosis or occlusion is a frequent complication and necessitates reintervention [4.10]. CDS, especially in the power mode, has an important role in postinterventional follow-up.

Figure 43.4 shows a patent stent. Intimal hyperplasia often produces a constriction (⬊) at the center of the stent.

Figure 43.5 illustrates a stenosis, which typically develops at the site where the stent **(b)** enters the hepatic vein. The most reliable signs of stenosis are an abrupt velocity change (see spectra **a** and **b**) in the course of the stent and direct visualization of the narrowed site [4.10].

The Doppler spectrum in **Fig. 43.6** does not reflect flow signals but the artifactual vibrations of an occluded stent (⬇), evidenced by the typical symmetrical pattern of spikes.

Intrahepatic tumors

CDS can be very helpful in the differentiation of indeterminate vascular and solid masses in the liver. Adenomas, focal nodular hyperplasia (FNH), and hemangiomas that display typical features can be distinguished from malignant tumors. The inability to detect flow in a homogeneous hyperechoic mass, despite proper equipment settings, suggests a hemangioma [4.11, 4.12]. This diagnosis can be reinforced by demonstrating additional flow characteristics with the aid of contrast agents (see below).

The use of contrast agents

While the use of Doppler and power-Doppler imaging has improved the differential diagnosis of intrahepatic lesions over conventional B-mode imaging in recent years [22], problem cases still exist even for experienced examiners:

First, some hepatic lesions located deep in the abdomen and in very obese patients can be scanned only at an unfavorable Doppler angle, which can greatly limit the accuracy of the finding. Second, the very slow flows that are commonly encountered, especially in small tumors, produce inadequate frequency shifts. Third, motion artifacts can be extremely difficult to avoid in some areas of the liver due to the transmission of cardiac movements to the hepatic parenchyma.

Ultrasound contrast agents, combined with modified scanning techniques, can provide crucial help in problem cases such as these. They produce strong intravascular signal enhancement (see pp. 107) that can improve the detection of even slow flows in smaller tumor vessels.

Several different enhancement phases are observed following the bolus injection of a contrast agent. These phases can vary somewhat according to the individual circulatory status of the patient **(Table 44.1)**.

Enhancement phases following intravenous contrast administration	
Early arterial:	15-25 seconds postinjection
Arterial:	20-30 seconds postinjection
Portal:	40-100 seconds postinjection
Late venous:	110-180 seconds postinjection

Table 44.1 [Modified from 4.23]

Benign hepatic lesions: FNH and adenoma

Benign hepatic lesions, unlike malignant lesions, do not contain increased pathologic shunt connections. As a result, benign lesions still show contrast enhancement even in the late venous phase. This occurs with focal nodular hyperplasia (FNH) and hemangioma. FNH most commonly affects women who are regular oral contraceptive users. Hepatic adenomas can display almost identical features in the B-mode image, and differentiation often requires histologic examination. Both color-flow and power Doppler **(Fig. 44.3a, b)** can clearly demonstrate the typical flow pattern of FNH, which is an important aid to differential diagnosis.

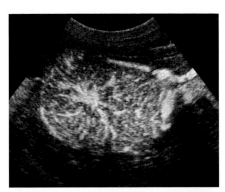

Fig. 44.2 (Dr. Dietrich, University of Frankfurt)

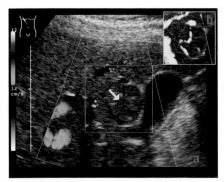

Fig. 44.3a, b

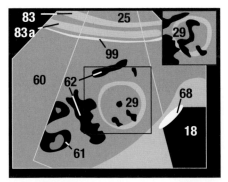

Fig. 44.3c

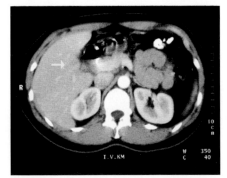

Fig. 44.3d

The vascular plexus in FNH emanates radially from a central artery (⭢) and exhibits centrifugal flow [4.12], giving rise to a "spoked wheel" pattern **(Figs. 44.2 and 45.2 c)**. FNH and adenoma can both cause symptoms due to expansile growth or intrahepatic hemorrhage and may therefore require surgical resection. On CT scans, FNH and adenomas are defined most clearly in the early arterial phase of enhancement (⟹ **Fig. 44.3d)**. During the parenchymal phase, they appear hyperechoic or isoechoic to the surrounding liver tissue.

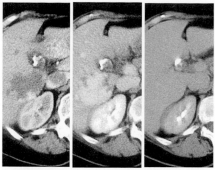

Fig. 45.1

Hepatic hemangiomas

Unlike FNH, hemangiomas are vascularized in a peripheral-to-central pattern **(Fig. 45.2b-e)**. During the arterial phase **(Fig. 45.2c)** the outer portions of the lesion enhance while the center remains hypoechoic. The central portions become increasingly echogenic during the subsequent portal phase **(Fig. 45.2d)**, and the entire lesion appears hyperechoic in the late venous phase **(Fig. 45.2e)**. This progressive, peripheral-to-central pattern of enhancement, called also the "iris diaphragm" sign, is often somewhat irregular and is typical of hepatic hemangiomas. It is also appreciated in CT scans **(Fig. 45.1)**.

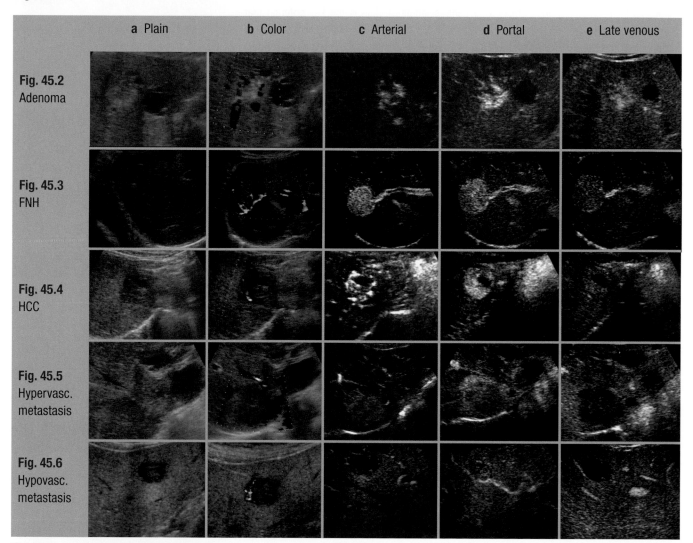

	a Plain	**b** Color	**c** Arterial	**d** Portal	**e** Late venous
Fig. 45.2 Adenoma					
Fig. 45.3 FNH					
Fig. 45.4 HCC					
Fig. 45.5 Hypervasc. metastasis					
Fig. 45.6 Hypovasc. metastasis					

Fig. 45.2 - 45.6 Characteristics of focal hepatic lesions (by S. Rossi, M.D.)

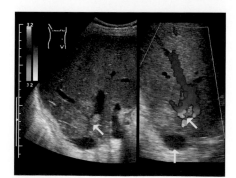

Fig. 45.7

Hepatocellular carcinoma (HCC)

The detection of intra- and peritumoral arterial Doppler signals, vascular cutoffs, vascular invasion, corkscrew-like configurations, and increased arteriovenous shunts are generally regarded as malignant criteria in CDS [4.12, 4.13]. Hepatocellular carcinomas (HCC) generally show nonhomogeneous signal enhancement in the arterial phase following contrast administration **(Fig. 45.4c)**. They remain hyperechoic during the portal phase **(Fig. 45.4d)** and then usually become isoechoic to healthy liver parenchyma in the late venous phase **(Fig. 45.4e;** [23]). **Figure 45.7** shows an HCC located at the confluence of the hepatic veins. Portions of the tumor (↖) have invaded the obstructed middle hepatic vein. That vessel is stenosed just proximal to its junction with the IVC (⇑), posing a risk of Budd-Chiari syndrome.

Hepatic metastases

Hepatic metastases may be hypo- or hypervascular. Although the location of the primary tumor cannot be reliably determined from the vascularization pattern [4.18], it has been found that certain primary tumors are associated with typical degrees of vascularity. Neuroendocrine primary tumors such as C-cell carcinoma of the thyroid gland or carcinoid tend to seed hypervascular metastases **(Fig. 45.5)**, whereas colorectal primary tumors tend to have hypovascular metastases **(Fig. 45.6)**.

During the arterial phase after contrast injection, metastases usually show only slight peripheral enhancement with conventional scanning technique, depending on their degree of vascularity **(Figs. 45.5c** and **45.6c)**. They generally remain hypoechoic to the liver parenchyma in the late venous phase **(Figs. 45.5e** and **45.6e)** or may become isoechoic [4.23]. This low echogenicity in the late venous phase after contrast administration is the key criterion that differentiates metastases from the benign hepatic lesions previously described. What accounts for this? A distinguishing characteristic of hepatic metastases is their tendency to form numerous pathologic arteriovenous shunts. This can explain why contrast agents tend to clear more rapidly from hepatic metastases than from normal liver parenchyma, producing a relatively hypoechoic appearance of the metastases in the late phase of contrast perfusion.

Signs typical of hepatic metastases are irregular perfusion patterns, corkscrew-like vascular configurations **(Fig. 46.1)**, and the presence of increased arteriovenous shunts. Because of these shunts, it takes only about 20 seconds, rather than the usual 40 seconds, for the contrast agent to appear in the hepatic veins. Often the clinical presentation will aid in differentiating between HCC and metastasis: patients with an HCC often present with hepatic cirrhosis, chronic hepatitis, and/or an elevated serum AFP (alpha-fetoprotein). This combination is found more rarely in patients with hepatic metastases from other primary tumors.

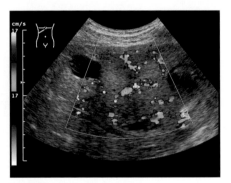

Fig. 46.1

Special scanning techniques

When scanning is performed with a low mechanical index (MI ~ 0.1), often combined with the phase inversion technique, fewer microbubbles are destroyed at once during initial bolus transit. This prolongs the contrast enhancement. At the same time, the use of a low MI decreases the sensitivity of the examination. For example, when a low MI is used, posterior acoustic enhancement is no longer an effective criterion for distinguishing a cyst from other hypoechoic lesions. In some cases posterior acoustic enhancement will reappear only after the MI has been increased to the "normal" range of 1.0 to 2.0.

The intermittent transmission of only 2 ultrasound pulses per second, rather than 15 ("intermittent harmonic imaging"), makes it possible to detect even small capillaries, since the longer interpulse delays result in less microbubble destruction, making a higher concentration of bubbles available for capillary signal enhancement when the delayed pulses enter the tissue [4.24].

With this technique of intermittent pulse transmission at a low MI, even hypovascular hepatic metastases appear hyperechoic during the early arterial phase (the first 5-10 seconds of contrast transit) [4.24], creating a visible distinction between the early arterial and arterial phases of enhancement.

Rule of thumb for the differential diagnosis of hepatic lesions

The use of contrast agents permits the following differentiation: Lesions that show more prolonged signal enhancement are more likely to be benign, while metastases and HCC often appear hypoechoic to the surrounding liver parenchyma even in the late venous phase [4.23].

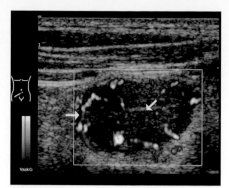

Abb. 47.1a

Inflammatory bowel diseases

Despite the difficult scanning conditions in the gastrointestinal tract, a number of pathologic conditions can be diagnosed with ultrasound. The B-mode image alone can suggest an inflammatory process by showing exudation and thickening of the bowel wall. The detection of hypervascularity (⇒ **Fig.47.1**) can further support the suspicion of a chronic or acute inflammatory bowel disease. **Figure 47.1** a shows a cross-sectional view of a stenosed terminal ileum (✍) due to inflammatory wall thickening in Crohn disease. The corresponding fluoroscopic view (**Fig.47.1b**, small bowel contrast study using the Sellink technique) demonstrates a long segment of residual lumen. Acute enteritis and radiation enteritis (**Fig.47.2**) are also characterized by nonspecific hypervascularity (⇐), leading to an increased flow velocity and increased volume flow in the SMA [4.15]. Appendicitis also presents with nonspecific hypervascularity in the thickened and inflamed bowel wall.

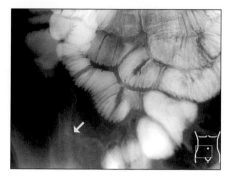

Fig. 47.1b

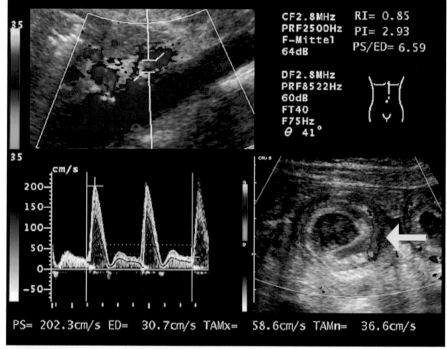

Fig. 47.2

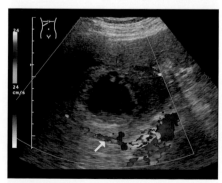

Fig. 47.3a

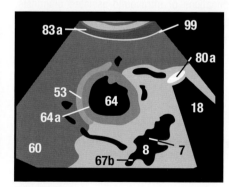

Fig. 47.3b

Figure 47.3 shows a perforated gallbladder **(64)** in a patient with severe underlying cholecystitis. The wall **(64a)** shows typical pronounced hypervascularity with a long visualized segment of the cystic artery (↗). Extraluminal gallbladder fluid **(53)** has eroded the proper hepatic artery **(67b)**, creating a false aneurysm **(8)** (see p.39).

Critical Evaluation

CDS is a powerful noninvasive study that has varying roles and capabilities in the different organs and vascular systems of the abdomen. Usually the liver is easily accessible to ultrasonography even under difficult clinical conditions, and specific indications have been established for the evaluation of focal and diffuse changes in the liver parenchyma and hepatic vascular systems. Indeed, CDS has become the imaging procedure of first choice for the diagnosis and surveillance of portal hypertension and for the planning and follow-up of TIPSS insertion. CDS allows the noninvasive measurement of flow velocity and volume flow, reliably detects complications such as stenosis and occlusion, and is useful in selecting cases for revision by interventional angiography.

CDS can be used for the postoperative follow-up of liver transplantations to confirm organ perfusion. In contrast to its routine use in renal transplants, however, there is no standard cut-off value for a resistance increase that would permit a diagnosis of hepatic allograft rejection [4.16, 4.17].

The characterization of focal hepatic lesions based on degree of vascularity and vascular architecture remains a controversial issue. Several malignant criteria are already known that permit a more accurate diagnosis of focal hepatic lesions [4.12]. The use of ultrasound contrast agents promises to improve the detection of vascularity and time-varying perfusion patterns for this type of application.

In studies of abdominal vessels, CDS is used mainly for the screening and surveillance of aneurysms. Complementary modalities such as CT, MRI, and contrast angiography may be necessary for therapeutic and preoperative planning. CDS has also become an established screening method in chronic intestinal ischemia.

The ability of CDS to detect increased vascularity in inflammatory diseases such as appendicitis and cholecystitis has further advanced the capabilities of diagnostic ultrasound.

An experienced examiner can devise specialized, nonstandard indications for CDS by using a transducer with high spatial resolution. Certain characteristics of the method can be limiting, however. For example, considerable time may be needed to complete a reliable study. Moreover, the examiner-dependence of CDS is particularly high in the abdomen because of the variable acoustic conditions. With advances in electronic data processing, however, imaging results will continue to improve, providing increasingly more detailed and easy-to-interpret images like those produced by the panoramic SieScape technique and 3-D reconstructions. The presentation and reporting of findings still pose a problem, however.

Tissue harmonic imaging is a new modality that can be used in problem cases to improve imaging when abdominal scanning conditions are poor. The use of many different ultrasound contrast agents has greatly improved the applications of ultrasound-assisted diagnosis, follow-up, and intervention, particularly in patients with hepatic lesions. Thus, CDS continues to provide a noninvasive imaging procedure with a high development potential that is sure to find further applications in abdominal imaging.

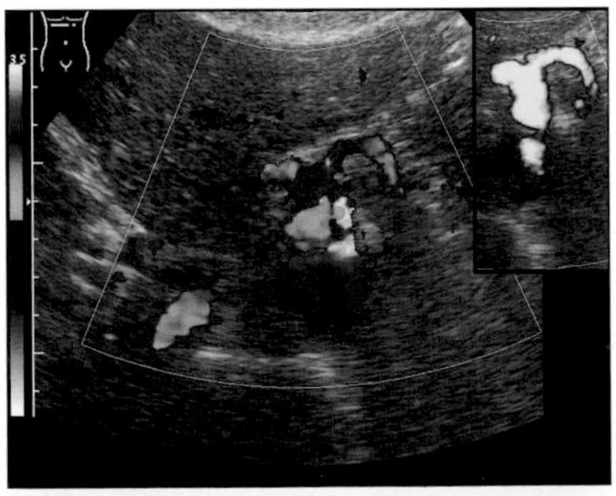

Fig. 48.1

Q

Quiz – **Take the following quiz to test your knowledge:**

Conduct a step-by-step interpretation of the two pathologic images on the right, based on the following questions:

1. What planes are imaged?
2. What organs and landmarks help to establish orientation?
3. What display modes were used?
4. What vessels are shown and what is the flow direction?
5. Do you see any characteristic flow phenomena?
   Are the flow data within normal limits?
6. What strikes you as unusual compared with normal findings?
7. What is your presumptive diagnosis?

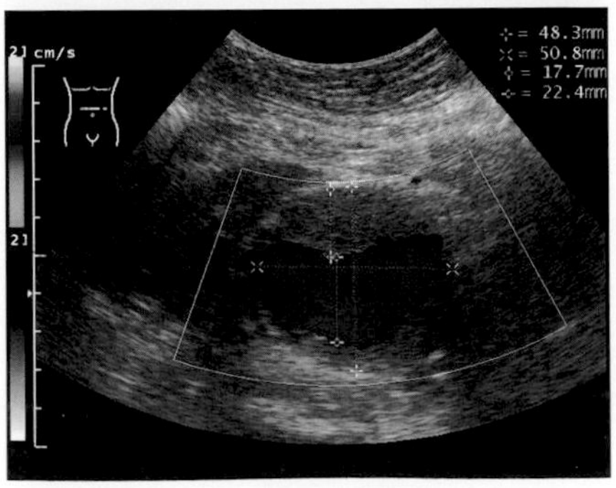

Fig. 48.2

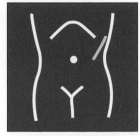

Markus Hollenbeck
Gerald Antoch

Introduction

Color duplex scanning (CDS) has added an important dimension to renal ultrasound studies. CDS can provide conclusive evidence of renal artery stenosis (RAS), and examiners need no longer be content with offering a diagnosis of "vascular atrophic kidney." Doppler ultrasound can detect pathologic changes even before they have led to structural tissue alterations.

Renal allografts can be visualized particularly well with ultrasound owing to their superficial location in the iliac fossa. Allograft rejection can be detected at an early stage, and problems with the graft artery and principal veins can be accurately diagnosed. CDS can replace practically all radionuclide and angiographic studies in renal allograft evaluations.

CDS has also gained increasing importance in urologic studies. With its rapid availability, it has become important in the differential diagnosis of acute scrotal disorders and can facilitate the decision for operative or conservative treatment. It also provides crucial etiologic information in the assessment of erectile dysfunction. Traditional, more invasive diagnostic procedures are increasingly superseded by CDS.

Native kidneys: examination technique and normal findings

The patient is examined in a fasting state. Because the renal arteries are deeply situated, we use a low-frequency transducer operating at 2.0 to 3.5 MHz.

Anatomy and transducer position

The right renal artery **(124a)** branches from the aorta **(30)** at about the 10-o'clock position, arising slightly below the origin of the superior mesenteric artery. It curves posteriorly and passes behind the IVC **(76)** on its way to the right renal hilum **(Fig. 50.1a)**. The left renal artery **(124b)** arises from the aorta at about the 4-o'clock position, usually on the same level as the right artery. It can be traced for approximately 3 cm from the aorta to the hilum. It is more difficult to visualize than the right renal artery, as it is more frequently obscured by gas in overlying loops of small bowel **(80b)**.

Angle-corrected velocity measurements are taken at five points along the course of the main renal arteries. Normal peak velocities range from 50 to 160 cm/s.

Accessory renal arteries are present in 20% of patients, and the aorta should therefore be scanned cranial and caudal to the renal artery origins so that any additional renal arteries can be identified.

The renal arteries can be visualized in an oblique coronal longitudinal section **(Fig. 50.1b)** with the transducer placed on the right midclavicular line, or they can be imaged in an abdominal transverse section **(Fig. 50.1a)**.

The best view is obtained by positioning the transducer just above the midway point between the xiphoid process and the umbilicus. If bowel gas obscures visualization of the aorta at this location, move the transducer up to the subxiphoid level and angle it downward, or scan from a more caudal level and angle the transducer upward. The best acoustic window will vary depending on the bowel gas distribution at the time of the examination.

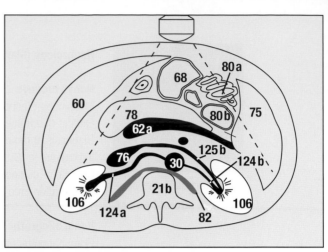

Fig. 50.1a

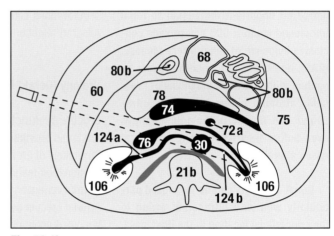

Fig. 50.1b

Normal findings

When the origin of the right renal artery **(124a)** is imaged with color flow, it is common to find an area of color inversion (⇑) in the curved vessel. The relatively dark color shades **(Fig. 50.2a)** distinguish this normal phenomenon from the bright color shift that is caused by aliasing due to proximal renal artery stenosis. Note also the normal appearance of the arterial lumen. **Figure 50.2b** shows the normal left renal artery **(124b)** arising from the aorta **(30)** anterior to the spinal column **(21b)**. The arterial spectrum displays a steep systolic peak (⇲), a clear spectral window (⇓), and a smooth downslope to diastole (⇖). The apparent discrepancy in flow velocities between the right and left arteries is due merely to different scale selection in each example. Actually there is very little difference between the peak systolic velocities (90 vs. 98 cm/s).

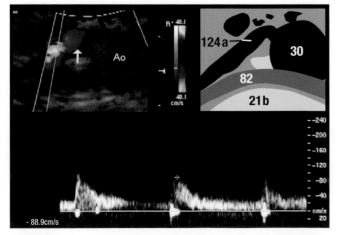

Fig. 50.2a

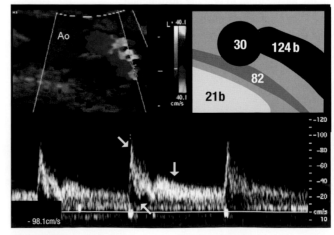

Fig. 50.2b

Examination technique and normal findings

Oblique coronal longitudinal scans are obtained in the left lateral decubitus position. The transducer is oriented longitudinally and placed in the midclavicular line (**Fig. 51.1a**). It is angled until the vena cava is demonstrated in longitudinal section. If bowel gas obscures visualization, the transducer should be moved over the skin and angled accordingly until a satisfactory acoustic window is found. The aorta (**30c**) is visualized "behind" the vena cava (**76**). The right renal artery (**124a**) passes directly toward the transducer from the aorta (**Fig. 51.1b**). The flow directly toward the transducer produces a large Doppler frequency shift, yielding conspicuous color flow and a well-defined Doppler spectrum. The left renal artery (**124b**) courses away from the transducer. This projection of the renal arteries is best for determining whether one or more polar arteries are present.

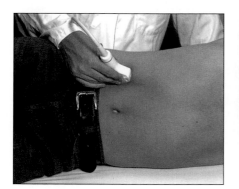

Fig. 51.1a

Fig. 51.1b

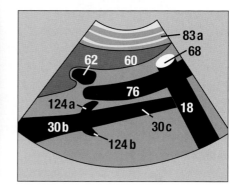

Fig. 51.1c

Doppler spectra from the intrarenal interlobar arteries

First, the kidneys are optimally visualized in the B-mode image in the left and right lateral decubitus positions. This can also be done in a standard supine position in most patients. After obtaining an optimum B-mode view, activate color flow and duplex and measure successive RI values in the proximal, middle, and distal thirds of at least three interlobar arteries. In a healthy subject, the RI values will show only minimal differences within one kidney and between the kidneys. A mean value is calculated from the resistance indices for each kidney.

The RI values measured in healthy subjects show a significant dependence on age and the area sampled. The values in the main artery are higher in the hilar region (0.65 ± 0.17) than in the more distal smaller arteries, and they are lowest in the interlobar arteries (0.54 ± 0.20). Comparable values are obtained only when arteries of equal order are sampled. The best sampling sites are the segmental and interlobar arteries (**Table 51.2**), as these vessels are easy to find at the junction of the renal pelvis and parenchyma. They usually pass directly toward the transducer and produce a high Doppler frequency shift, resulting in good-quality color flow and spectral images.

Age-related change in the renal RI

RI values are also age-dependent: they are higher in elderly patients. Renal blood flow is more "pulsatile" in older patients, because the windkessel function declines while renal flow resistance increases due to interstitial fibrosis. Normal age-dependent RI values for the interlobar arteries are shown in **Table 51.2**.

In **Figure 51.3**, comparison of the Doppler spectra of a 42-year-old patient (**a**) and a 79-year-old patient (**b**) vividly demonstrates the age-related change in flow pattern. The RI of the younger patient, at 0.61, is significantly lower than the RI of 0.84 measured in the older patient.

Normal RI values in the interlobar arteries of hypertensive patients [5.1]		
Age (years)	m	m ± 2 SD
< 20	0.567	0.523–0.611
21–30	0.573	0.528–0.618
31–40	0.588	0.546–0.630
41–50	0.618	0.561–0.675
51–60	0.668	0.603–0.733
61–70	0.732	0.649–0.815
71–80	0.781	0.707–0.855
> 81	0.832	

Table 51.2

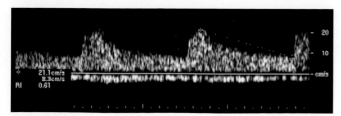

Fig. 51.3a

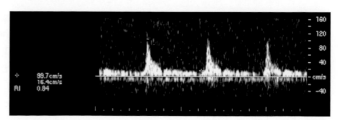

Fig. 51.3b

Factors that influence renal perfusion

Age is by no means the only factor that affects intrarenal resistance indices. **Table 52.1** lists additional intrarenal and extrarenal factors that must be taken into account when interpreting RI values. It should be noted that these factors are far more common in transplanted kidneys than in native kidneys, and that when bilateral, they do not adversely affect the side-to-side comparison of RI values in the diagnosis of RAS (see below).

Cause of increased flow resistance	Pathophysiology
Acute renal failure	Swelling of kidney due to interstitial edema, tubulo-juxtaglomerular feedback with mesangial contraction and constriction of afferent vessels
Obstruction of renal pelvis	Interstitial edema due to back-filtration of intratubular fluid into the interstitium
Extrarenal compression	Interstitial pressure increased due to subcapsular hematoma or other mass
Low diastolic blood pressure	Deficient propulsive force in diastole (e.g., due to severe aortic valve insufficiency)
Bradycardia	Scant flow at the end of prolonged diastole
Interstitial scarring	Interstitial fibrosis or small-artery sclerosis leads to rarefaction of terminal arterial branches with an increase in flow resistance
Acute rejection	Interstitial rejection: enlargement of allograft due to interstitial infiltration by lymphocytes Vascular rejection: increased resistance due to narrowing of small intrarenal arteries
Cyclosporin A toxicity	Cyclosporin A has a vasoconstricting effect on the afferent vessels

Table 52.1

Diagnosis of renal artery stenosis (RAS)

The narrowing of an artery lumen generally leads to flow acceleration. While less than 50% stenosis causes only slight flow acceleration, the velocity increases sharply with a higher-grade stenosis and then declines sharply as the stenosis nears 100% **(Fig. 52.2)**. Because of this flow acceleration, stenoses are encoded in bright colors in CDS. High-resolution scanning under favorable conditions can demonstrate turbulence **(5)** in the form of yellow-green mosaic patterns downstream from the stenosis. A stenosis cannot be confidently diagnosed with color flow alone, however. Spectral traces should always be acquired in suspicious areas so that the flow velocities can be determined.

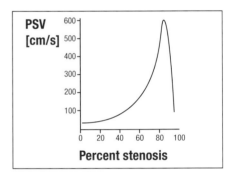

Fig. 52.2

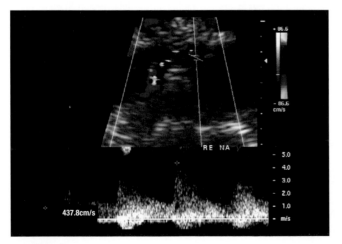

Fig. 52.3a

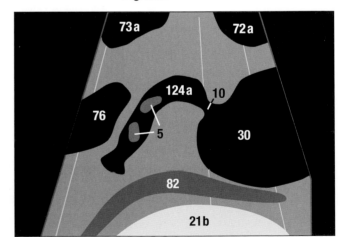

Fig. 52.3b

An experienced examiner (more than 500 renal-artery color duplex examinations) using modern equipment can demonstrate 70-90% of the renal arteries. The visualization of accessory renal arteries is more difficult and succeeds in approximately 20-50% of cases [5.2]. An experienced sonographer can complete the examination in 30-45 min.

The typical color duplex features of a high-grade RAS **(Fig. 52.3)** are its flow acceleration greater than 200 cm/s (here: 438 cm/s) and poststenotic turbulence **(5)** in the lumen of the affected renal artery **(124a)**.

Situations in which CDS is indicated:
Hypertension in a patient under 30 years of age
More than 1.5cm right-left discrepancy in renal size
Diastolic blood pressure > 105 mm Hg despite triple antihypertensive regimen, especially in patients with severe generalized atherosclerosis
Creatinine rise while on treatment with ACE inhibitors or AT-1-receptor antagonists

Table 53.1

Criteria for diagnosing RAS
PSV > 200 cm /s (Direct criterion)
Right-left difference in RI values > 0.05 (Indirect criteria)
→ RAS in the kidney with the lower RI
RI on each side is below the age-normal range → bilateral RAS (Indirect criteria)
→ Acceleration time >70 ms (measured in the segmental arteries)

Table 53.2

Indications for CDS of the renal arteries

CDS is indicated only if there is definite clinical suspicion of renovascular hypertension. It makes no sense for every patient with hypertensive disease to undergo CDS; this would generate an inordinate number of false-positive results. At least one of the suspicious signs of RAS listed in **Table 53.1** should be present before CDS is performed.

Criteria for diagnosing renal artery stenosis

A direct sign of RAS is a measured flow velocity higher than 200 cm/sec in a main renal artery. The indirect signs of RAS are based on the fact that every stenosis greater than 70% causes flow disturbances in the poststenotic vascular segment. The poststenotic systolic peaks are rounded (✎), here showing a PSV of only 8 cm/s **(Fig. 53.3a)**. This leads to decreased (!!) RI values in the poststenotic vessel [5.22]. Comparison with the contralateral kidney **(Fig. 53.3b)** shows a normal-appearing waveform in one of the right interlobar arteries.

A prolonged acceleration time (AT) may also be measured past the stenosis. The AT is the time from the start of systolic acceleration to the point where the waveform flattens (arrows in **Fig. 53.5**). By looking at these indirect signs of stenosis, evidence for the presence of RAS can be gained even in cases where the renal arteries themselves cannot be visualized due to overlying gas. **Table 53.2** lists the essential criteria for diagnosing RAS. The condition should be diagnosed when at least one of the criteria is met.

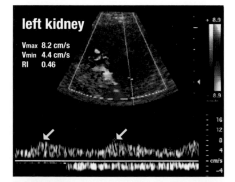

Fig. 53.3a

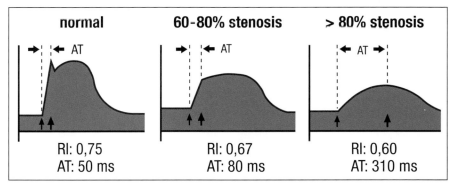

Fig. 53.5 acceleration time (AT)

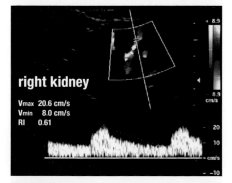

Fig. 53.3b

In patients with absolute arrhythmia, the PSV can vary considerably in different pulse cycles due to variations in the stroke volume of different cardiac contractions **(Fig. 53.4)**. Although the color-flow quality on each side was poor in this case due to obesity, it is clear that the peak flow velocity is increased to approximately 395 cm/s in the right renal artery **(Fig. 53.4a)** and to approximately 410 cm/s in the left renal artery **(Fig. 53.4b)**. For comparison, **Fig. 53.4c** shows how the amplitude-based power Doppler mode can provide a better color-encoded image of the proximal renal arteries. The strength of this technique lies in the improved visualization of vascular segments that run horizontal to the beam axis, despite the absence of directional and velocity information.

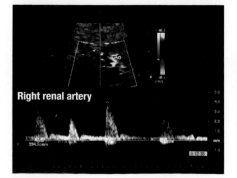

Fig. 53.4a

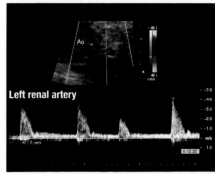

Fig. 53.4b

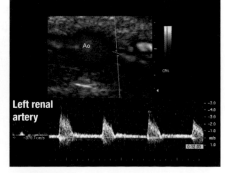

Fig. 53.4c

Renal allografts – examination technique

The examination technique for renal allografts must allow for the fact that the graft artery and vein are more tortuous than in a native kidney due to the location of the transplant and the configuration of the surgical anastomoses. The examination is usually easier than in native kidneys because the allograft is close to the skin. Also, the number of polar arteries has already been documented in the operative report. More than 95% of all known graft arteries can be completely visualized with modern equipment.

Graft artery stenosis

The renal allograft is a functioning solitary kidney that may undergo considerable compensatory hypertrophy. Because renal blood flow depends strongly on renal function, we cannot define a specific cutoff point for diagnosing RAS as we can in native kidneys. In a hypertrophic, well-functioning renal allograft, the flow velocity may be higher than 250 cm/s throughout the nonstenosed artery. But in the case of chronic allograft dysfunction with a decrease in renal size, regional flow acceleration to 200 cm/s may indicate significant RAS if the flow velocities in other portions of the main artery are only 50 cm/s.

Thus, a localized flow acceleration that is more than 2.5 times the prestenotic or far poststenotic velocity (e.g., 260 cm/s vs. 100 cm/s) provides a direct criterion for stenosis in an allograft renal artery. The sensitivity and specificity of CDS exceed 90% in the detection of stenoses [5.3]. There are no indirect signs of RAS as in native kidneys, because the right and left sides cannot be compared and because the flow resistance depends on many other factors (see **Table 52.1**).

Figure 54.1 shows the effect of sample volume position **(11)** on measured peak velocity in a high-grade stenosis of the allograft artery **(124c)** at its anastomosis with the external iliac artery **(127a)**. The flow velocity decreases from 450 cm/s within the stenosis **(Fig. 54.1a)** to approximately 80 cm/s distal to the stenosis **(Fig. 54.1c)**.

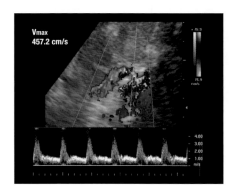

Fig. 54.1a

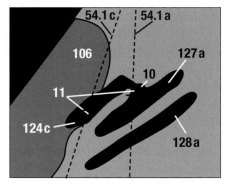

Fig. 54.1b

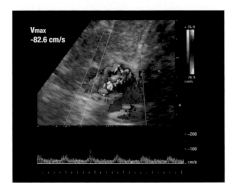

Fig. 54.1c

Graft vein thrombosis

Complete thrombosis of the allograft vein is recognized by an inability to demonstrate intrarenal veins in the hilum and by pathognomonic bidirectional flow in the intrarenal arteries.

This bidirectional flow pattern results from the maximal rise in flow resistance caused by the complete renal vein thrombosis. Blood that flows into the renal arteries during systole flows back out again in diastole. Net blood flow through the kidney is reduced to zero, and the average flow velocity over one cardiac cycle is equal to zero! This means that in the Doppler spectrum, the areas above the baseline during the brief periods of systolic inflow (✓) equal the areas of diastolic reverse flow (⇑) below the baseline **(Fig. 54.2)**. This pattern is so specific for allograft vein thrombosis that it warrants a recommendation for immediate surgical revision without any additional studies.

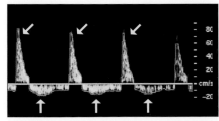

Fig. 54.2

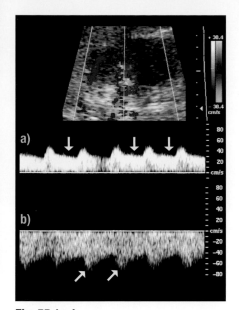

Fig. 55.1a, b

Arteriovenous fistulas in renal allografts

The most frequent cause is renal biopsy. The fistula often appears on color Doppler as a non-specific mosaic pattern of reds and blues. The diagnosis is confirmed if the feeding arteries show decreased flow resistance with an increase in diastolic flow (⬇) **(Fig. 55.1a)** and the draining veins show a pulsatile pattern (➶) of accelerated flow **(Fig. 55.1b)**. Patients with a large AV fistula are at higher risk for hemorrhagic complications during repeat renal biopsy.

In the example shown, CDS demonstrates a large-caliber interlobar artery and vein. The RI of the feeding artery **(a)** is 0.50, compared with approximately 0.80 in other regions of the allograft. The venous spectrum **(b)** shows a strongly pulsatile flow pattern that is not found in other interlobar veins.

Allograft rejection

CDS is of particular value in detecting early signs of renal allograft rejection. An increase in flow resistance is a very early sign of rejection, preceding a deterioration of renal function (serum creatinine) by approximately two days. Increased resistance is not a specific sign of rejection, since various intrarenal and extrarenal factors can increase the PI or RI of a renal allograft (see **Table 52.1**).

Figure 55.2a illustrates a normally perfused renal allograft on the 10th postoperative day. During the days preceding the study, the RI declined from 0.84 to 0.75, paralleling the resolution of acute postischemic renal failure and the fall in serum creatinine levels. CDS was repeated on the 13th postoperative day **(Fig. 55.2b)**, at which time the serum creatinine was a constant 1.5 mg/dl while the RI had increased to 1.00. The elevation of intraparenchymal pressure caused a cessation of end-diastolic blood flow (⬃). The clinical suspicion of acute allograft rejection was confirmed histologically by renal biopsy. High-dose steroid therapy was initiated, and the RI values subsequently declined.

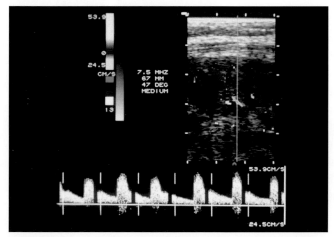

Fig. 55.2a

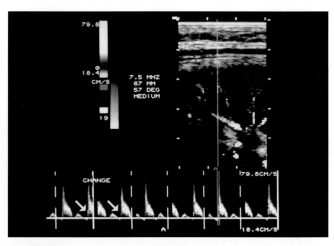

Fig. 55.2b

When a high RI is found on just one occasion, it cannot be determined whether the increase is due to acute postischemic renal failure, for example, or to allograft rejection. A rising resistance index noted in serial examinations (every 3-4 days) is a more reliable indicator of rejection than a single value. While the resistance index and pulsatility index are of approximately equal importance in all other studies, the daily increase in PI is a better indicator of rejection than an increase in RI, because the PI in patients with constant zero diastolic flow reflects small changes in systolic inflow better than the RI (see p. 12).

When we observe an increase in PI, we proceed with allograft biopsy at once unless the overall clinical course mitigates against rejection. Early biopsy in rejection allows for early histologic confirmation and treatment.

If an elevated PI does not decline in response to rejection therapy, the therapy may be inadequate. We recommend performing a repeat biopsy in these cases to assess the need for further immunosuppression.

Erectile dysfunction

Anatomic orientation

The penis consists of two corpora cavernosa **(95)** and the corpus spongiosum **(95a)**, which surrounds the urethra **(104)** and forms the bulb proximally and the glans distally. The smooth muscle of the corpora cavernosa forms endothelium-lined cavities (sinusoids) that communicate with the arterial vascular system of the penis. Both corpora cavernosa are invested by a tough fascial layer called the tunica albuginea **(105) (Fig. 56.1)**.

The penis derives its blood supply from two penile arteries **(94)**, which arise as terminal branches from the internal pudendal arteries. Past the origin of the penile bulbar artery **(100)**, the penile artery of each side devides into the urethral artery **(103)**, the superficial dorsal artery **(94b)** and the deep penile artery **(94a)** of the corpus cavernosum. Within the corpus cavernosum, the deep penile artery gives off numerous helicine arteries **(102)**, which open into the cavernous sinusoids **(Fig. 56.2a)**. **Figure 56.2b** shows both deep penile arteries (⇑ + ⇓) with their helicine arteries (⇐) as they are defined by power Doppler (see p. 106). The corpora cavernosa are drained by subtunical venules that empty into the deep dorsal vein of the penis **(96a)**.

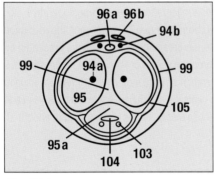

Fig. 56.1

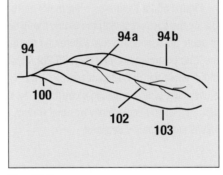

Fig. 56.2a

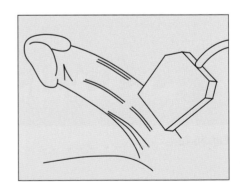

Fig. 56.2b

Physiology of erection

When the penis is flaccid, the smooth muscle of the corpora cavernosa is in a state of maximal contraction. The peripheral resistance is high, and the penis receives scant arterial flow. At the onset of erection, the cavernosal smooth muscle relaxes in a neurotransmitter-mediated response, thereby lowering the resistance in the corpora cavernosa and causing the afferent arteries to dilate. This results in increased arterial blood flow and an expansion of penile volume (the tumescent phase). As the tough tunica albuginea **(105)** is poorly distensible, the increasing blood volume compresses the venules located between the blood-filled sinusoids and the tunica. Venous outflow ceases, and the penis becomes rigid.

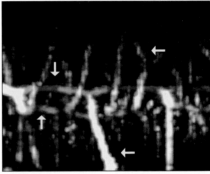

Fig. 56.3a

Examination technique and normal findings

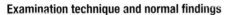

The patient is examined supine with a high-frequency linear-array transducer. The deep penile arteries are scanned in longitudinal and transverse section from the ventral base of the penis **(Fig. 56.3a, b)**, and their Doppler spectra are recorded. The measurements are standardized to the basal region of the penis, because as the vessels taper distally in caliber, it is normal for their peak systolic velocity (PSV) to decline.

Examination of the penile vessels in the preinjection state (before the intracavenous injection of an erection-inducing drug) is optional, since the arterial flow patterns in the flaccid penis are basically the same in healthy subjects as in patients with erectile dysfunction [5.5].

The PSV in the non-erect penis is only 5-20 cm/s, consistent with the high penile resistance. There is no detectable antegrade diastolic flow (EDV = 0 cm/s). The resistance index (RI) equals 1.0 **(Fig. 57.1a)**. A minimum pulse repetition frequency and wall filter should be used in order to obtain good color-flow images and adequate spectra.

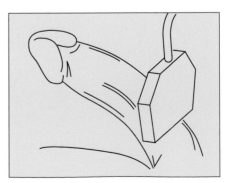

Fig. 56.3b

An elastic tourniquet is placed on the base of the penis, followed by the injection of a vasoactive agent that induces smooth-muscle relaxation to expand the cavernous sinusoids and produce arterial dilatation. The needle is inserted at the dorsal base of the penis, and the agent is injected into the corpus cavernosum on one side; anastomoses between the corpora cavernosa will distribute the agent to both sides. Prostaglandin E1 (10-20 mg) has become the preferred agent over papaverine or a papaverine-phentolamine mixture owing to the reduced risk of prolonged erection. After the prostaglandin has been administered and the tourniquet removed, both deep penile arteries are alternately scanned while the PSV, EDV, and RI are continuously determined. The postinjection arterial and sinusoidal dilatation causes the PSV to increase above 40 cm/s [5.7, 5.8]. Due to the massive decrease in peripheral resistance, the diastolic flow velocities increase markedly to more than 10 cm/s (⇩ in **Fig. 57.1b**) while the RI falls below 0.7 **(Fig. 57.1b)**.

As the sinusoids become increasingly engorged, a renewed increase in penile resistance occurs. As a consequence the peak systolic velocity declines with the level of flow still remaining significantly higher than in the flaccid state. The diastolic waveform approaches the baseline and finally dips below the baseline throughout diastole (⇩ in **Fig. 57.1c**) as a sign of bidirectional flow in the deep penile arteries. The RI rises above 1.0 **(Fig. 57.1c)**. The PSV, EDV, and RI should be continuously measured and an adequate examination time (approximately 30 min) should be maintained as the course of blood flow changes can vary strongly among different individuals [5.6].

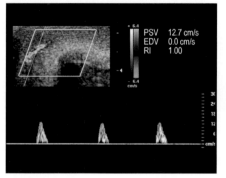

Fig. 57.1a

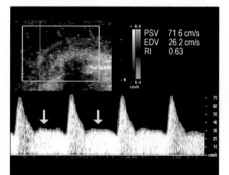

Fig. 57.1b

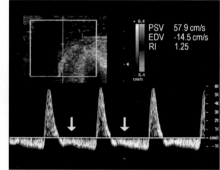

Fig. 57.1c

The dorsal penile arteries are of minor importance for satisfactory erectile function, and so it is unnecessary to scan these vessels [5.9]. After all spectra have been recorded, a systematic color-flow survey of the penis is carried out to detect any anomalies in the course of the arterial vascular tree. At the end of the examination, the patient should be informed that, in case of a pharmacologically induced prolonged erection, he needs to see a urologist within 4 hours to avoid the risk of irreversible loss of erectile function.

Normal variants

Figure 57.2 is from a patient with congenital hypoplasia **(111)** of the left deep penile artery in the basal region. Portions of the corpus cavernosum **(95)** located distally to the hypoplasia in this patient are supplied by an anastomosis from the dorsal penile artery **(94b)** (the anastomosis is not shown here). On finding this type of anomaly, the sonographer should also examine the superficial arteries and assess the functional competence of the anastomoses.

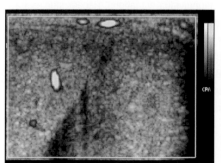

Fig. 57.2a

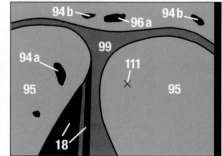

Fig. 57.2b

Arterial erectile dysfunction

While congenital anomalies in the penile vascular tree can be clearly identified in the color-flow image, the diagnosis of arterial erectile dysfunction is based mainly on a Doppler spectral analysis of the deep penile arteries. In patients with arterial stenoses in the lesser pelvis, scans obtained after prostaglandin injection will demonstrate a lower-than-normal peak systolic velocity during the tumescent phase (**Fig. 58.1**). A PSV < 25 cm/s in the deep penile artery is definitely pathologic. Values in the range of 25-35 cm/s are classified as borderline [5.10]. The systolic upslope is markedly flattened, resulting in a broadened, undulating spectral waveform (↘ ↗ in **Fig. 58.1**). Unlike the PSV, the degree of arterial dilatation after pharmacologic stimulation has proven to be an unreliable parameter in the evaluation of erectile dysfunction [5.7, 5.10] and is no longer a part of routine ultrasound studies.

Subtotal pharmacologic erections are common due to the subjectively unpleasant aspects of the postinjection examination. Before vascular erectile dysfunction is diagnosed, the patient should therefore be given the opportunity for 2-3 min of self-stimulation while the examiner leaves the room. This is followed by rescanning of the penile vessels and evaluation of the Doppler spectra.

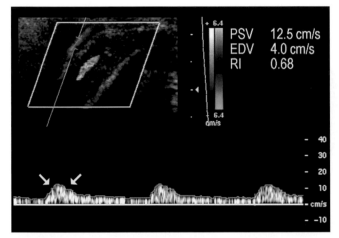

Fig. 58.1

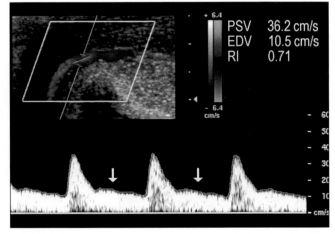

Fig. 58.2

Venous erectile dysfunction

Venous erectile dysfunction is detected indirectly by analyzing Doppler spectra recorded from the deep penile arteries. Normal compression of the draining venules by the increasing blood volume is manifested by a decrease of forward diastolic flow, or even reverse flow, in the deep penile artery. The resistance index reaches values higher than 1.0 (see **Fig. 57.1c**).

If venous incompetence is present, the rise in intracavernous pressure and increase in resistance are greatly reduced due to constant venous leakage from the corpora cavernosa. Antegrade diastolic flow persists, and the resistance index does not rise above 1.0. **Figure 58.2** shows typical color duplex findings with persistent end-diastolic velocities (EDV) of 10.5cm/s (↓) and a RI of 0.71 approximately 30 min after pharmacologic stimulation and repeated self-stimulation. Clinically there was no more than a subtotal erection.

The detection of venous flow in the penis does not always signify venous incompetence, because some degree of venous drainage from the glans and corpus cavernosum is present even in full erection. It is difficult to define normal values for end-diastolic flow velocities and resistance indices, because both parameters show great interindividual variations. Recent studies have shown that even the persistence of antegrade end-diastolic velocities in the deep penile arteries may be associated with normal venous function [5.11, 5.12]. Despite this limitation, CDS can provide important evidence of venous incompetence, which can then be further investigated by cavernosometry and cavernosography. **Figure 58.3** shows the cavernosogram of a patient with venous erectile dysfunction. The arrows (↙↘) indicate pathologic drainage of the intracavernously administered contrast medium through veins of the lesser pelvis.

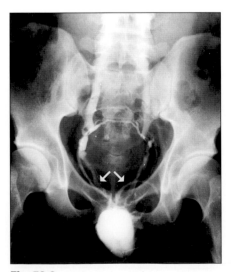

Fig. 58.3

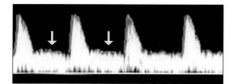

Fig. 59.1

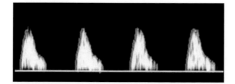

Fig. 59.2 a

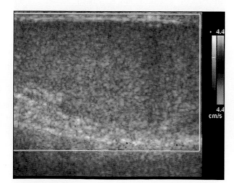

Fig. 59.2 b

Sonography of the scrotum

Blood supply to the testis

The testis derives its blood supply from the testicular artery **(98)**, which arises from the abdominal aorta below the renal arteries. It descends with the cremasteric artery **(98a)** and the deferential artery **(98b)** through the inguinal canal and, on reaching the scrotum, gives off branches to supply the epididymis. The main trunk of the testicular artery enters the testicle in the area of the mediastinum testis. It spreads out below the tunica albuginea as the capsular artery **(101)** and distributes branches toward the mediastinum testis. These branches course in the testicular septa and form recurrent branches **(98c)** that supply the seminiferous tubules **(Fig. 59.1)**. The testis is drained by the pampiniform plexus, the veins of which converge to form the testicular vein after passing through the inguinal canal. The testicular vein on the right side empties into the inferior vena cava, and that on the left side drains into the left renal vein. The vessels of both the arterial and venous systems are interconnected by multiple anastomoses.

Examination technique and normal findings

The testis is examined in the supine position using a high-frequency linear-array transducer. As blood flow velocities in normal testicular tissue are low, the scanner should be adjusted to detect low frequency shifts. Each testis and epididymis are imaged in the longitudinal and transverse axes. Size, shape, and echogenicity should be evaluated and compared with the opposite side. The normal testicular parenchyma has a homogeneous internal echo pattern and is surrounded by an echogenic capsule (tunica albuginea). Color flow should demonstrate equal perfusion of both testes. A typical Doppler spectrum from the testicular artery and intratesticular arteries shows a biphasic flow pattern with an antegrade diastolic component (⇓ in **Fig. 59.2 a**) as a sign of low peripheral resistance. Sampling the supratesticular arteries between the superficial inguinal ring and testis yields spectra that do not have this diastolic flow component. These are arterial spectra from the cremasteric and deferential arteries **(Fig. 59.2 b)**, which represent a vascular territory with high peripheral resistance [5.13].

It is sometimes difficult to demonstrate arterial inflow in prepubescent boys due to the small testicular volume and low blood flow velocities [5.14]. The color duplex image of the normal epididymis demonstrates very little blood flow. Therefore it is important to assess perfusion by comparing the right and left sides.

The acute scrotum

The main entities to be considered in the differential diagnosis of acute testicular pain are testicular torsion and epididymitis. Swift diagnosis is important, as a twisted testicle will suffer irreversible damage within 4-6 hours [5.14]. The imaging procedure of choice in such an emergency is CDS.

Testicular torsion

The most important sonographically detectable change in the initial hours after testicular torsion is absent or decreased perfusion of the symptomatic side compared with the opposite side [5.15, 5.16]. **Figure 59.3 a** shows the color duplex findings in a patient with acute left testicular pain in contrast to the normal perfusion of the asymptomatic right testis **(Fig. 59.3 b, c)**.

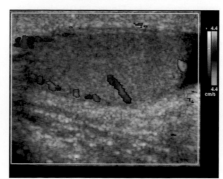

Fig. 59.3 a

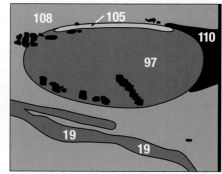

Fig. 59.3 b

Fig. 59.3 c

The degree of hypoperfusion on the affected side depends on the duration and severity of the torsion. With subtotal torsion (<360°), some residual perfusion of the affected testis can often be detected [5.15, 5.16]. Venous obstruction precedes arterial obstruction in less severe cases, with the result that arterial spectra can still be recorded from the affected testis while venous spectra cannot. In these cases it is important to suspect testicular torsion and proceed with immediate surgical exposure to avoid hemorrhagic infarction of the tissue [5.17]. As the torsion continuous, an increase in blood flow in the peritesticular tissue and scrotal skin can be shown and should not be mistaken for testicular perfusion.

Unlike color flow, it takes 6–8hours for changes to appear in the B-mode image. The testis appears enlarged, and its parenchyma becomes nonhomogeneous and echopenic. The scrotal skin is thickened on the affected side, and a hydrocele may develop. If spontaneous detorsion occurs, the ischemic interval may be followed by a compensatory increase in testicular perfusion, and it can be difficult to differentiate the torsion from epididymo-orchitis. Like testicular torsion, hydatid torsion (torsion of the appendix testis or appendix epididymis) is associated with testicular pain of acute onset. At ultrasound the twisted appendix usually appears more echogenic than the adjacent testicular and epididymal parenchyma. Color duplex can demonstrate reactive inflammation of adjacent portions of the testis and epididymis as an increase in blood flow.

Epididymitis

The B-mode imaging of epididymitis shows an enlarged epididymis with a non-homogeneous internal echo pattern. If the inflammation involves the testis (epididymo-orchitis), adjacent testicular areas also appear nonhomogeneous. CDS shows markedly increased perfusion of the affected areas compared with the opposite side. **Figure 60.1** demonstrates the color flow features of inflammation involving the head of the epididymis (**97a**), a reactive hydrocele (**110**), and thickening of the scrotal wall (**53**).

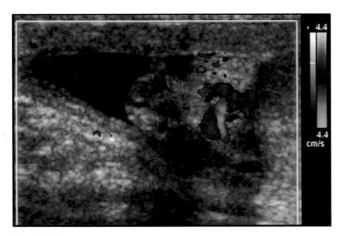

Fig. 60.1a

Fig. 60.1b

The Doppler spectrum also shows characteristic changes on the affected side. Normally the epididymis shows only a small amount of diastolic flow (⬇ in **Fig. 60.2 a**). Inflammation lowers the vascular resistance in the epididymis, leading to a marked increase in diastolic flow. The resistance index is decreased in relation to the asymptomatic side. **Figure 60.2 b** shows the Doppler spectrum from the symptomatic side in a patient with acute scrotal pain; diastolic blood flow is markedly increased compared with the asymptomatic side (**Fig. 60.2 a**) while the RI is reduced to 0.59. As the resistance indices show large interindividual variations, the findings should be compared with the opposite side in the same patient rather than with standard normal values. If complications arise (abscess formation, hemorrhagic infarction), it can be difficult to distinguish inflammation from traumatic changes or tumors (see p. 61).

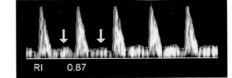

Fig. 60.2 a

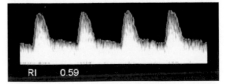

Fig. 60.2 b

Testicular tumors

Testicular tumors appear sonographically as nonhomogeneous masses in the testicular region. Local calcifications appear as hyperechoic foci with a posterior acoustic shadow, while intratumoral necrotic areas appear hypoechoic. CDS has only an adjunctive role in the diagnosis of testicular tumors because even though the detection of localized hyperperfusion due to pathologic blood vessels supports the suspicion of a tumor, the absence of this hypervascularity does not exclude a tumor. **Figure 61.1** shows the sonographic appearance of a testicular tumor with hyperperfused areas, intratesticular calcifications **(3)**, and necrotic components **(109)**.

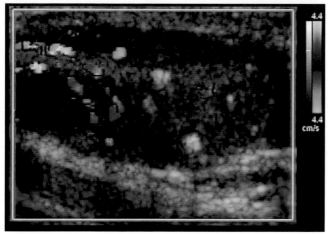

Fig. 61.1a

Fig. 61.1b

Varicocele

The patient should be examined in both the supine and standing positions, because standing creates a higher hydrostatic pressure that distends the tortuous venous structures and helps to detect them more easily. B-mode ultrasound supports the diagnosis of a varicocele by demonstrating the dilated veins of the pampiniform plexus **(107)** as wormlike anechoic structures. **Figure 61.2** illustrates the appearance of a varicocele at the upper pole of the testis **(97)**. By raising the intra-abdominal pressure, a Valsalva maneuver can reverse flow in the testicular vein and the veins of the pampiniform plexus, producing a color inversion in the color-flow image and a direction change in relation to the spectral baseline. The dilated tortuous veins persist for a time following treatment, but color imaging no longer detects blood flow even in response to a Valsalva maneuver.

The plexus dilatations are generally extratesticular, but a large varicocele may also affect intratesticular veins [5.18]. The differentiation of idiopathic from symptomatic varicocele relies on abdominal ultrasound, giving particular attention to masses involving the kidneys and retroperitoneum.

The advantage of color duplex over clinical examination alone lies in the ability of CDS to detect subclinical varicoceles. When used in regular follow-ups after varicocele treatment, CDS can detect a recurrence of the disease at an early stage.

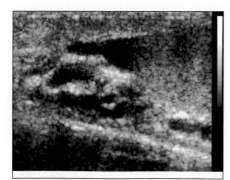

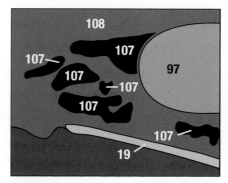

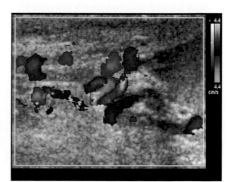

Fig. 61.2 a

Fig. 61.2 b

Fig. 61.2 c

Critical evaluation

An experienced examiner (more than 500 renal-artery color duplex examinations) using modern equipment in a fasted patient can define 85% of all renal arteries. This figure takes into account any polar arteries, but the visualization of these arteries is a weakness of CDS in renovascular studies. A polar artery that arises at a low level from the iliac artery is almost always missed.

RAS can be diagnosed with 85-90% sensitivity and specificity using both direct and indirect criteria [5.4]. Whenever RAS is detected by duplex sonography or is suspected clinically, DSA should be performed **(Fig. 62.1 a)** and facilities should be available to proceed with dilatation if required. An RI value less than 0.80 in the nonstenosed contralateral kidney is considered a favorable prognostic sign.

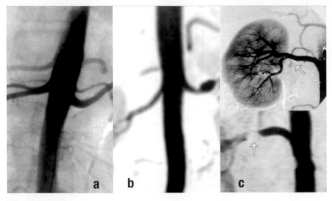

Fig. 62.1

There is hope in such cases that correcting the stenosis will improve renal function and blood pressure [5.20].

Useful follow-up studies besides DSA, especially after percutaneous transluminal angioplasty, are the noninvasive procedures of CDS and MR angiography (MRA, **Fig. 62.1 b**). MRA, however, is of limited value following the angiographically guided placement of a vascular clip (✏) or stent, as these devices will produce signal voids (⇧) within the magnetic field **(Fig. 62.1c)**. In these cases MRA can furnish only indirect information on restenosis based on the differential timing of contrast appearance in both kidneys.

In some respects, CDS is superior to angiography. Besides the ability of CDS to measure volume flow, a stenosis can be causally related to, say, compression from a hematoma on the basis of color duplex findings. When the volume flow is known, the hemodynamic significance of a stenosis can be evaluated better than with angiography. CDS can be used in these cases for the surveillance of moderate to higher-grade stenoses with good flow characteristics. Prospective and randomized studies [5.21] have shown that regular CDS examinations at 6-month intervals with prophylactic dilatations of >50% stenoses lead to a significant decline in the rate of shunt occlusion and in costs.

In patients with erectile dysfunction, CDS is superior to conventional Doppler in its ability to evaluate penile morphology and also quantify blood flow velocities. While CDS is accurate in the diagnosis of arteriogenic erectile dysfunction, the diagnosis of venous incompetence is difficult due to a lack of normal values for the EDV and RI. So if venous leak is suspected as the cause of erectile dysfunction, ultrasound should be supplemented by cavernosometry and cavernosography.

Currently there is a debate as to the benefits and therapeutic implications of establishing the etiology of erectile dysfunction [5.19], because most patients respond well to intracavernous autoinjection therapy (ICAT) or oral medication, regardless of the underlying cause.

With its lack of invasiveness and convenience of use, CDS has replaced radionuclide imaging in the differential diagnosis of the acute scrotum and is now considered the method of choice among imaging procedures. CDS, however, does not always yield unequivocal findings, and in such cases it cannot eliminate the need for immediate surgical exposure of the testis. CDS is superior to B-mode imaging in the evaluation of testicular trauma and the detection of varicocele. For tumor diagnosis and for the localization of undescended testes, conventional ultrasound or even MRI should be used.

Quiz – Take the following quiz to test your knowledge: (the answers are at the end of the book)

1. How can you detect unilateral RAS when the main vessels are obscured by overlying gas?
2. What is the cutoff flow velocity in a main renal artery that would indicate RAS?
3. How would you interpret an RI of 0.50 in the interlobar arteries of both kidneys in an 80-year-old patient?
4. How would you interpret the color-flow and spectral findings in the right renal artery in **Fig. 62.2 a** and **b**?
5. **Figure 62.3** shows the sonographic appearance of the left testis and epididymis in a 35-year-old man with acute left-sided scrotal pain. On physical examination, the left epididymis is enlarged and markedly tender. The right epididymis is clinically and sonographically normal. What diagnosis do these findings suggest?
6. A 54-year-old man gave a 6-month history of an increasing, painless swelling in the right scrotum. On palpation, the epididymis felt hard and markedly enlarged. No abnormalities were found in the testis itself. What diagnosis does **Fig. 62.4** suggest, and what differential diagnoses

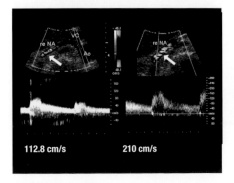

Fig. 62.2 a and **b**

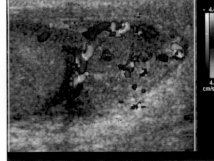

Fig. 62.3

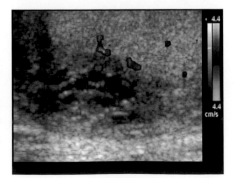

Fig. 62.4

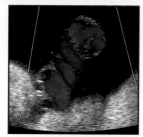

Tatjana Reihs
Matthias Hofer

Obstetrics

The obstetric use of CDS is described for specific vascular territories:

Introduction

Color duplex sonography (CDS) has become an established tool in obstetrics, particularly in the surveillance of high-risk pregnancies. Doppler examination is an important adjunct to gray-scale imaging if there is suspicion of intrauterine growth retardation (IUGR), pregnancy-induced hypertension (PIH), preeclampsia, or a fetal anomaly. Other indications for CDS are multiple pregnancy as well as chronic maternal diseases such as nephropathy or autoimmune disease, coagulation disorders, diabetes, and hypertension. Because color duplex operates at higher acoustic pressures than gray-scale imaging, it is wise to follow the ALARA principle ("as low as reasonably achievable") even though the exposure levels are generally below established limits [6.1].

A valid Doppler examination should be performed under conditions of maternal and fetal rest in the semilateral position to eliminate forced respiratory or body movements that could interfere with the examination. In interpreting the results, the examiner should take into account external influences such as caffeine, nicotine, and tocolytic agents. The Doppler parameters of primary interest are the absolute flow velocities, resistance index (RI), and pulsatility index (PI).

In contrast to obstetrics, the gynecologic applications of CDS, particularly in the diagnosis of pelvic masses, are still the object of numerous studies. Endovaginal CDS permits the detection of intratumoral blood vessels and can aid in the benign-malignant differentiation of gynecologic masses. CDS is also used in infertility patients for assessing tubal patency, monitoring follicular growth for in vitro fertilization (IVF), and detecting ectopic pregnancy.

Uterine artery

The uterine artery **(140)** is imaged lateral to the uterus **(141)** at the site where it crosses over the external iliac artery **(127a)** and external iliac vein **(128a)** **(Fig. 64.1a)**. It is important to recognize the uterine artery waveform **(Fig. 64.1a)**, which is influenced by gestational age and placental location. The waveform can be difficult to identify in obese patients and in late pregnancy. With a lateralized placental location, it is usual to find lower RI and PI values in the ipsilateral uterine artery than on the contralateral side of the placenta. Uterine contractions during labor reduce the blood supply to the intervillous space, leading to a rise in the Doppler indices. Conversely, heat application or β_2-sympathomimetics cause an increase in diastolic blood flow, and the indices are correspondingly low. The normal values for RI and PI are shown in **Figures 64.2 a** and **64.2 b**.

Normal RI values in the uterine artery

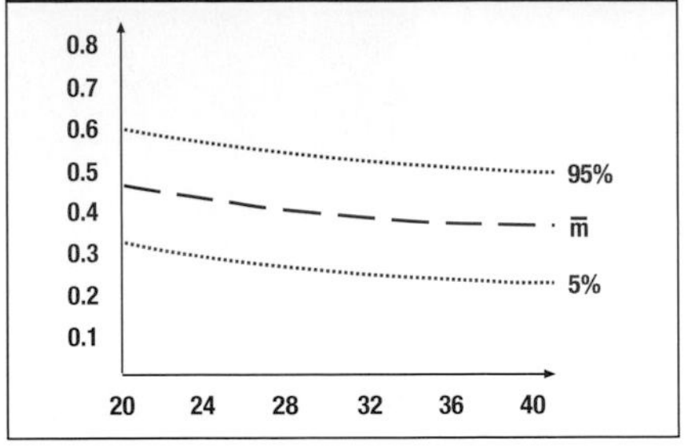

Table 64.2 a

Normal PI values in the uterine artery

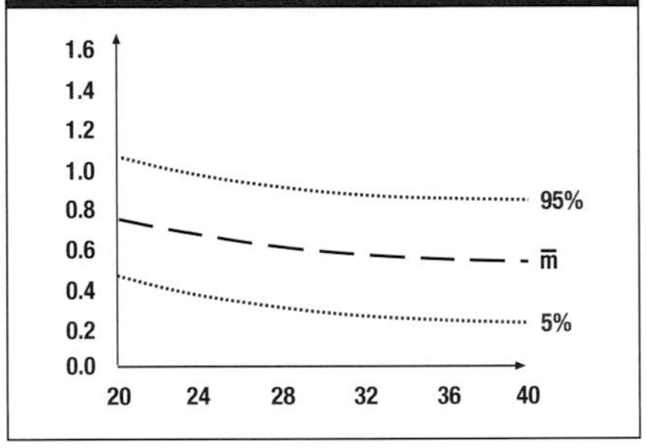

Table 64.2 b

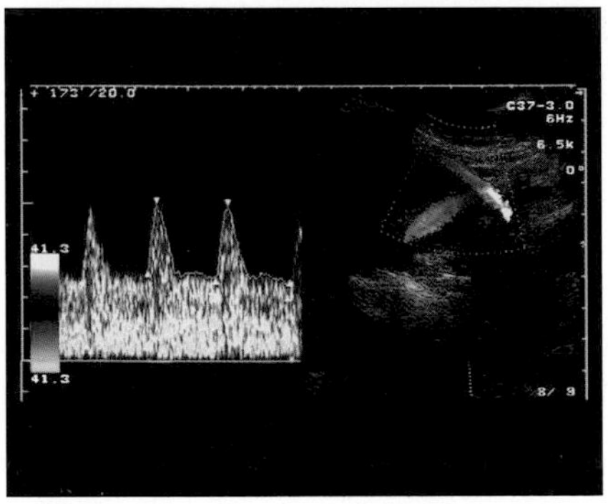

Fig. 64.1a

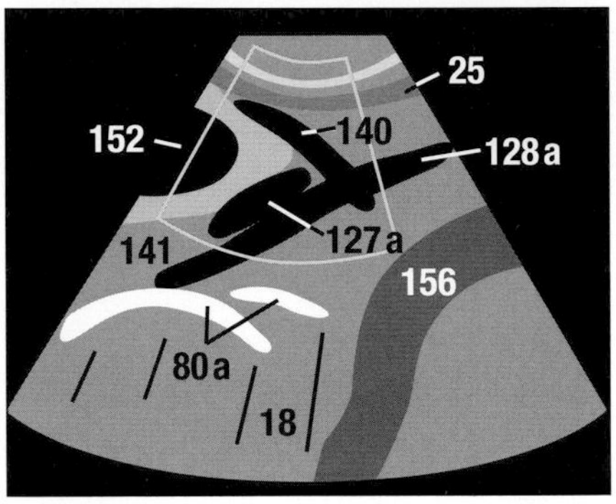

Fig. 64.1b

The uterine artery waveform during the first half of pregnancy shows a physiologic notch in early diastole (⇩ in **Fig.64.3a**), signifying high vascular resistance. This early diastolic notch should disappear by the 25th week of gestation.

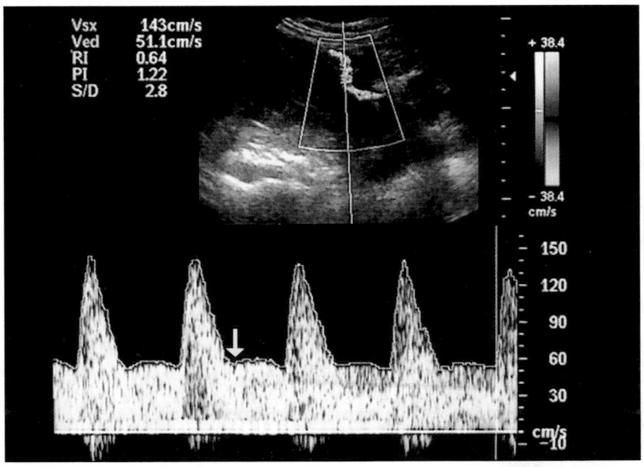

Fig. 64.3a

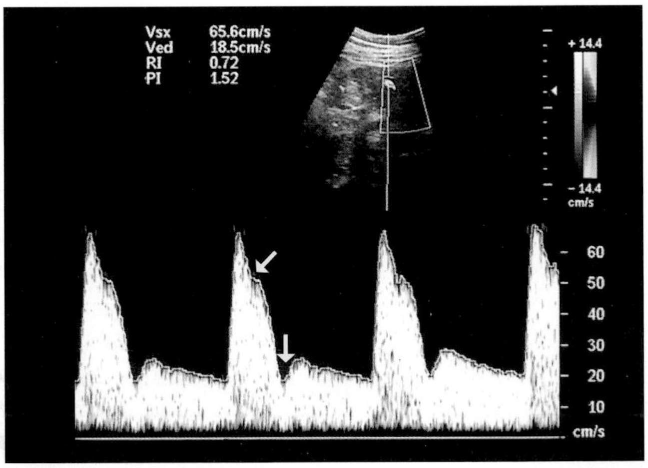

Fig. 64.3b

In a normal pregnancy, trophoblastic invasion destroys the elastic muscular wall of the spiral arteries, transforming them into wide channels and increasing the flow velocity in the uterine arteries. The persistence of a bilateral diastolic notch after 25 weeks' gestation is abnormal and is associated with an increased risk of preeclampsia, placental abruption, PIH, and IUGR. If the diastolic notch persists, aspirin therapy at a dose of 70-100 mg/day should be considered. If the patient is at risk by her prior history (e.g., hypertension, preeclampsia, placental insufficiency), aspirin therapy should be started in the 14th week of gestation. In cases of significant placental insufficiency, the postsystolic notch may be accompanied by a second, intrasystolic notch (⇙) that reflects an extremely high impedance in the placental vascular bed **(Fig. 64.3 b)**. Unlike the unilateral notch (see above), this phenomenon is considered a poor prognostic sign.

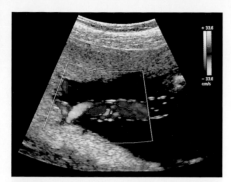

Fig. 65.1a

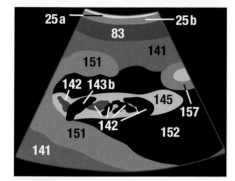

Fig. 65.1b

Umbilical artery

The two umbilical arteries **(142)** are approximately 50cm long and run through the amniotic cavity to the surface of the placenta **(151)**. There they divide into numerous chorionic plate vessels while the umbilical vein **(143)** runs in the opposite direction to the fetus. Generally the umbilical vessels are easy to visualize if the amniotic fluid volume is normal. Localization of the umbilical cord insertion **(Fig. 65.1)** is important for chorionic villus biopsy or fetal blood sampling (cordocentesis). A single umbilical artery (SUA), occurring in just 1% of all pregnancies, is associated with an increased risk of chromosome abnormalities, fetal malformations (approximately 20%), mortality, and prematurity **(Table 65.2)**. Localization of the site of the aplasia is an important guide in the search for fetal anomalies on the ipsilateral side. SUA is easily diagnosed by imaging the origin of the umbilical artery adjacent to the fetal urinary bladder **(144) (Fig. 65.3)**. The direction of blood flow in both vessels is easily assessed at that location. In the rare case of a twin pregnancy where there is suspicion of a TRAP sequence with severe reduction anomalies in the deprived fetus (acardia, anencephaly), CDS can detect retrograde perfusion of the umbilical arteries in the acardiac twin.

SUA is assiciated with an increased risk of
• Chromosome anomalies
• Malformations (ipsilateral side!)
• Premature birth
• Mortality

Table 65.2

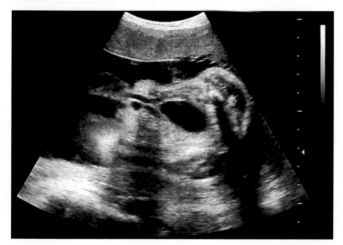

Fig. 65.3a

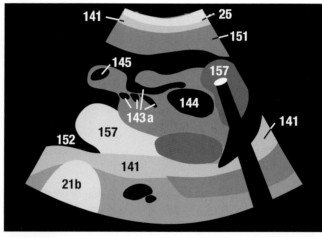

Fig. 65.3b

Short cord syndrome is a serious anomaly with a grave prognosis. The umbilical cord is extremely short or absent. This condition may be associated with absence of the fetal ventral abdominal wall.

Coiling of the umbilical cord around the neck is generally harmless **(Fig. 65.4)**. It occurs in approximately 50% of all births, is easily detected with CDS, and has no pathologic significance if the CTG is normal.

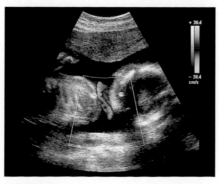

Fig. 65.4a

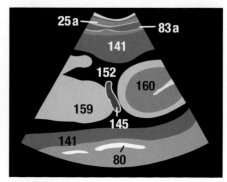

Fig. 65.4b

Umbilical artery

Diastolic flow cannot be detected in the umbilical arteries during the first ten weeks of gestation due to incomplete villous maturation. It is always detectable by the 15th week, however, and increases steadily as the pregnancy progresses **(Fig. 66.1a)**. The waveform of the umbilical artery **(142)** is significantly influenced by fetal respiratory and body movements and by changes in pressure relationships and heart rate. Because of the low resistance in the uteroplacental circulation, the RI and PI values on the placental side of the umbilical cord are generally lower than on the fetal side. The normal values for both indices are shown in **Figure 66.1b, c**.

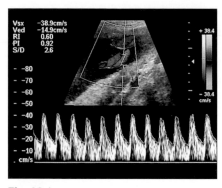

Fig. 66.1a

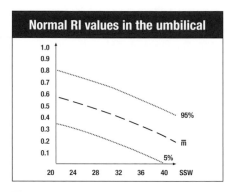

Fig. 66.1b

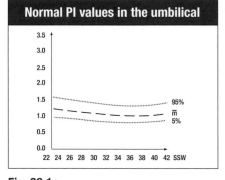

Fig. 66.1c

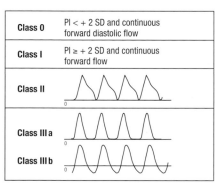

Table 66.2a

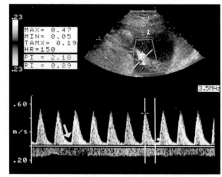

Fig. 66.2b

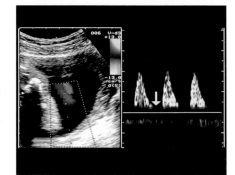

Fig. 66.2c

Several blood flow classes have been defined to describe spectral patterns observed in obstetric ultrasound **(Table 66.2a)**. Increasing pathologic significance is ascribed to a decrease in diastolic flow (in **Fig. 66.2b**, **class II**), an absence of diastolic flow (in **Fig. 66.2c**, **class IIIa**), or a reversal of diastolic flow (in **Fig. 66.3**, **class IIIb**). Classes IIIa and IIIb are associated with an approximately 45% increase in perinatal mortality rates **(Table 66.4)**. When pathology this severe is detected in the umbilical artery, the remaining fetal vessels should also be examined, including the middle cerebral artery (see p. 68), umbilical vein (see p. 69), and ductus venosus (see p. 70). A detailed evaluation to exclude fetal anomalies and chromosome abnormalities is also recommended in these cases.

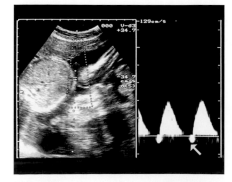

Fig. 66.3

Absence of diastolic flow and reverse flow in the umbilical artery		
Effect on perinatal outcome	**Mean value**	**Range**
Mortality (%)	45	17 - 100
Gestational age (weeks)	31.6	29 - 33
Birthweight (g)	1056	910 - 1481
SGA (%)	68	53 - 100
Cesarean section due to fetal distress (%)	73	24 - 100
Apgar score < 7 after 5 min (%)	26	7 - 69
Transfer to neonatal ICU (%)	84	77 - 97
Congenital anomalies (%)	10	0 - 24
Aneuploidy (%)	6.4	0 -18

Table 66.4 [6.1]

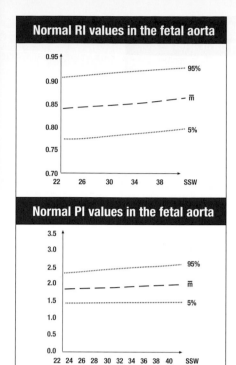

Normal RI values in the fetal aorta

Normal PI values in the fetal aorta

Fig. 67.1

Fetal Aorta

Doppler visualization and measurement of the aortic waveform is performed between the aortic arch **(30e)** and the origin of the renal arteries. Visualization of the vessel is often difficult due to an unfavorable beam angle or other problems. As a result, ultrasound scanning of the fetal aorta is not widely practiced at present, especially since the aortic waveform shows higher systolic-diastolic variability than the umbilical artery waveform. Diastolic flow cannot be detected until the second trimester and increases steadily during the course of pregnancy. Normal values for the aortic indices are shown in **Figure 67.1**.

It is normal for diastolic blood flow to decline at the end of pregnancy. This phenomenon is called the "term effect."

Normal values in the fetal aorta		
Peak systolic velocity	Mean value	Range
V_{max}	$\overline{m}$	$\overline{m} \pm 2\,SD$
25 weeks' gestation	80 cm/s	65 - 95 cm/s
37 weeks' gestation	100 cm/s	80 - 130 cm/s
> 39 weeks' gestation	90 cm/s	70 - 115 cm/s

Table 67.3

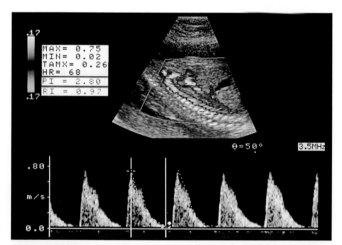

Fig. 67.2 a

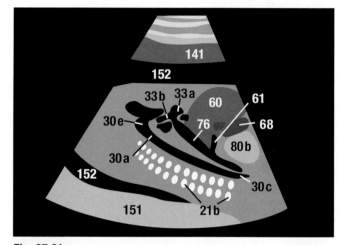

Fig. 67.2 b

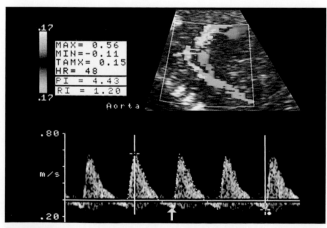

Fig. 67.4

An elevated peak velocity, on the other hand, may be a sign of fetal anemia. The normal values for peak systolic velocity [6.3] are shown in **Table 67.3**.

Significant intrauterine growth retardation (IUGR) is associated with a reduction of end-diastolic flow or even reversed flow (⇑) in the aorta **(Fig. 67.4)** as in the umbilical artery.

Fetal cerebral vessels: middle cerebral artery

The middle cerebral artery (MCA, **54b**) is the continuation of the intracranial carotid siphon (**40a**). It conveys approximately 40% of the volume flow from the circle of Willis to each cerebral hemisphere. It is best visualized in the sylvian fissure in a longitudinal sagittal section of the skull. The normal MCA spectrum is characterized by a high peak systolic velocity (✎) and a low diastolic velocity (⇧) (**Fig. 68.2 a**). The waveform is influenced, however, by fetal activity, pressure on the fetal skull, and intracranial masses. The normal RI (**Fig. 68.1a**) and PI (**Fig. 68.1b**) in the MCA decline steadily during the course of pregnancy and normally rise again at term.

During pregnancy the diastolic flow in the MCA is lower than in the umbilical artery. As a result, the cerebral vascular resistance (RI_{MCA}) is higher than the placental vascular resistance (RI_{PL}), and the cerebroplacental ratio (CPR = RI_{MCA}/RI_{PL}) in a normal pregnancy is greater than one. This index is a very sensitive predictor (80%) of fetal growth retardation:

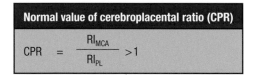

Normal value of cerebroplacental ratio (CPR)
$$CPR = \frac{RI_{MCA}}{RI_{PL}} > 1$$

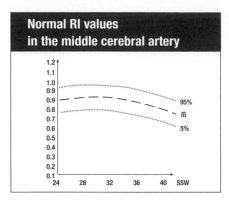

Normal RI values in the middle cerebral artery

Table 68.1a

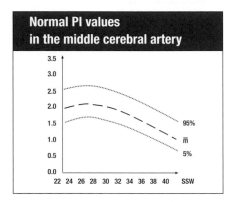

Normal PI values in the middle cerebral artery

Table 68.1b

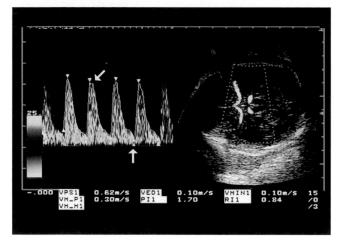

Fig. 68.2a

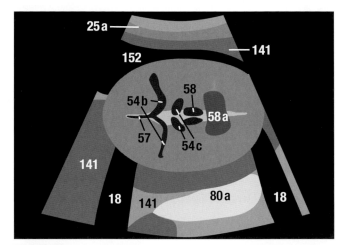

Fig. 68.2b

In cases of chronic fetal hypoxia, the blood volume in the fetal circulation is redistributed in favor of vitally important organs – the heart, kidneys, and brain. Vasodilatation of the MCA with an increase in diastolic flow and corresponding hyperperfusion is considered pathologic (**Fig. 68.3**). This "brain-sparing effect" is associated with an abnormal cerebroplacental ratio (< 1). If the hypoxia persists, however, the diastolic flow will return to a normal level. Presumably this reflects a terminal decompensation in the setting of acidemia or brain edema.

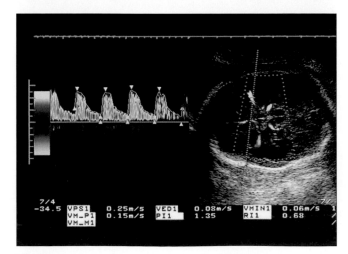

Fig. 68.3

Umbilical vein

The spectral waveform of the umbilical vein can be measured in its intra-abdominal, intra-hepatic, or extra-abdominal portion. The waveform typically shows a continuous low velocity of approximately 10-15 cm/s. But pulsatile flow may also occur in the umbilical vein **(143)** until about the 12th week of gestation due to a physiologic decrease in ventricular compliance. After 12 weeks, only respiratory and pressure-dependent variations are recorded **(Fig. 69.1a)**.

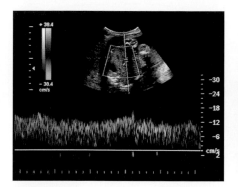

Fig. 69.1a

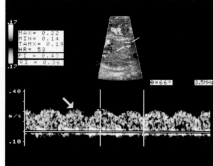

Fig. 69.1b

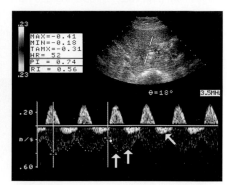

Fig. 69.1c

If there is a volume load on the heart as a result of congenital heart disease or fetofetal transfusion syndrome (FFTS), venous pulsations (↘) occur as a sign of cardiac decompensation or terminal placental insufficiency **(Fig. 69.1b)**. "Single pulsations" **(Fig. 69.1b)** that correlate with cardiac systole are distinguished from "double pulsations" **(Fig. 69.1c)**, which most likely result from significant cardiac insufficiency with reversed flow in the ductus venosus (see p.68). As a result, double pulsations are associated with increased perinatal mortality in approximately 55% of cases [6.10]. Both the arterial and venous waveforms shown in **Fig. 69.1c** are severely abnormal. Besides the double pulsations in the umbilical vein (⇑ ⇑), reverse flow (↖) is apparent in the umbilical artery (class III pattern, see p.64).

Inferior Vena Cava (IVC)

The typical waveform of the inferior vena cava **(IVC, 76)** is characterized by three points of flow acceleration: the S wave (↓) caused by movement of the valve plane during ventricular contraction, the D wave (↙) caused by passive ventricular filling, and the A wave (⇑) with physiologic flow reversal caused by atrial contraction **(Fig. 69.3a)**. Normal PI values for the IVC are shown in **Figure 69.2**. The A wave (reverse flow) is increased in the presence of right ventricular volume load or severe myocardial hypoxia.

**Normal PI values
in the inferior vena cava**

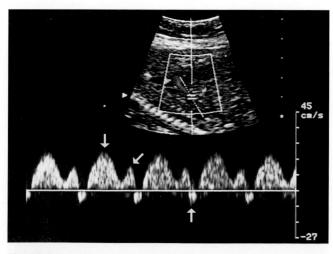

Table 69.2

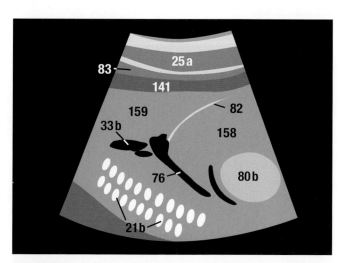

Fig. 69.3 a

Fig. 69.3 b

Ductus venosus

The ductus venosus **(DV, 146)** is easily identified by its turbulent flow pattern. The DV conveys approximately 50-60% (70% in fetal hypoxia) of the oxygen-rich blood from the placenta **(151)** to the right atrium via the umbilical vein **(143)** and inferior vena cava **(76)** and to the left atrium via the foramen ovale **(161)**. The schematic anatomy of these connections is shown in **Figure 70.1**. The ductus venosus is most easily visualized in a transverse scan through the fetal epigastrium **(Fig. 70.2)**. Three antegrade waves are visible in the ductus venosus waveform: the S wave (⬎) caused by ventricular contraction, the D wave (⬋) caused by passive ventricular filling, and the A wave (⬆) caused by atrial contraction **(Fig. 70.2)**. Normal PI values are shown in **Figure 70.3**.

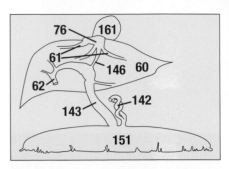

Fig. 70.1

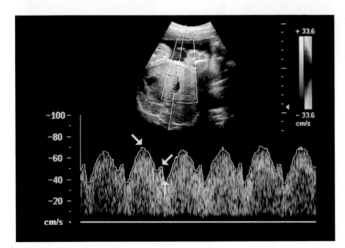

Fig. 70.2 a

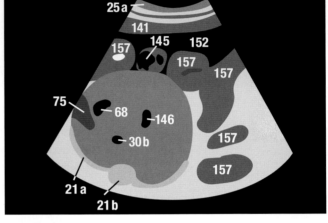

Fig. 70.2 b

All disturbances of cardiac hemodynamics that occur in association with tricuspid insufficiency lead to a steady decline in diastolic flow (⬇ **Fig. 70.4 a**) and ultimately to diastolic reverse flow (⬆) in the ductus venosus **(Fig. 70.4 b)**. These disturbances include arrhythmias, congenital defects, anemia, FFTS, and placental insufficiency. Reverse flow in the ductus venosus is again associated with an abnormal CTG and increased perinatal mortality [6.11].

Color duplex scanning of the ductus venosus is particularly important in cases of significant growth retardation with an abnormal arterial waveform. Doppler examination of the ductus venosus can be a very helpful study in cases where there is a steady deterioration of fetal condition and an impending risk of preterm delivery (< 35 weeks). If the flow in the DV is still "normal," the case can be managed by prophylaxis to promote fetal lung maturation. If reverse flow is found in the DV or if abnormal CTG changes arise, the fetus should be delivered by cesarean section.

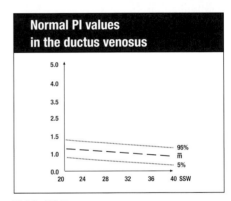

Table 70.3

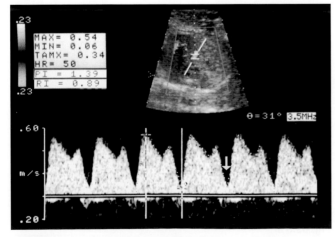

Fig. 70.4a

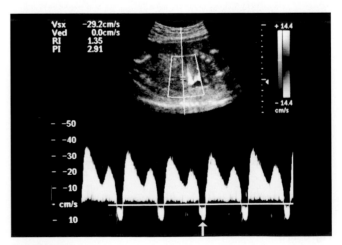

Fig. 70.4b

Ovaries

The optimum time for the color Doppler imaging of suspicious masses in the female reproductive tract is between days 3 and 10 of the menstrual cycle. During this phase of the cycle, vascular resistance is generally high due to estrogenic effects. This resistance declines markedly toward the middle of the cycle and remains low during the second half of the cycle. In postmenopausal women who are not on hormone replacement therapy, ovarian perfusion shows a high resistance pattern typically characterized by an early diastolic notch (✎) in the spectral waveform **(Fig. 71.1a)**. These flow patterns are characteristic of normal ovarian, uterine, and tubal perfusion.

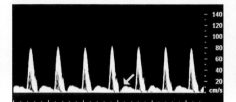

Fig. 71.1a

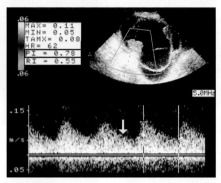

Fig. 71.1b

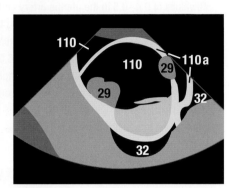

Fig. 71.1c

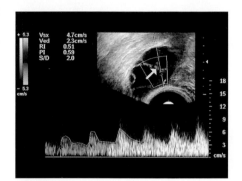

Fig. 71.2a

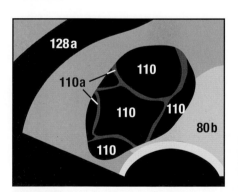

Fig. 71.2b

Malignant tumors, on the other hand, have a neovascularization pattern characterized by the absence of a muscle layer in the vessel walls and the development of sinusoids and numerous arteriovenous shunts. This creates a low resistance pattern with a PI less than 0.4 and RI less than 1.0. The velocity waveform shows a smooth downslope from systole to late diastole without a notch **(Fig. 71.1b** ⇓ **)**. The same neovascularization pattern can be seen in fast-growing, metabolically active benign tumors and also in follicular maturation, scar formation, and inflammatory processes.

Very low indices in the wall of a mature ovarian follicle or cyst **(110)** may be confused with similar findings in a mixed solid-cystic ovarian carcinoma. This fact complicates the benign-malignant differentiation of ovarian masses, especially in premenopausal women and in women on hormone replacement therapy. This uncertainty lends greater importance to factors such as the vascular distribution in a suspicious mass. For example, the detection of intraseptal **(110a)** vascularization (↗) in cystic ovarian masses **(Fig. 71.2a)** raises the index of suspicion for malignancy. Combining CDS with the ovarian tumor marker CA-125 can significantly improve the sensitivity of the method. Abnormal sonographic findings and elevated CA-125 levels are indicative of ovarian malignancy and warrant immediate open or laparoscopic exploration. The sonographic criteria for the classification of ovarian masses are shown in **Table 71.3**.

Classification of ovarian masses using B-mode ultrasound						
Mass	**Fluid**		**Inner margin**		**Interpretation**	
Unilocular	Clear	(0)	Smooth	(0)		
	Internal echoes	(1)	Irregular	(2)		
Multilocular	Clear	(1)	Smooth	(1)	**Ultrasound score**	
	Internal echoes	(1)	Irregular	(2)		
Cystic-solid	Clear	(1)	Smooth	(1)	≤ 2	**Benign**
	Internal echoes	(2)	Irregular	(2)		
Papillary growths	Suspicious	(1)	Definitive	(2)	3-4	**Equivocal**
Solid area	Homogeneous	(1)	Echogenic	(2)	> 4	**Suspicious**
Peritoneal fluid	Not present	(0)	Present	(1)		
Unilateral / bilateral	Unilateral	(0)	Bilateral	(1)		

Color duplex classification of ovarian masses					
Color Doppler		**Resistance index**		**Interpretation**	
– No detectable vessels	(0)		(0)		
– Uniform seperate vessels	(1)	> 0.40	(1)	**Color Doppler score**	
– Random vascular	(2)	< 0.40	(2)	≤ 2	**Benign**
If corpus luteum is suspected:				3-4	**Suspicious**
Repeat ultrasound in the proliferative phase of the next menstrual cycle					

Table 71.3, [6.8]

Uterus

The perfusion of the uterus **(141)** depends on the patient's reproductive age and whether she is receiving hormonal therapy. The normal spectral waveform of the uterine artery **(140)** is characterized by a high flow velocity, a resistance index (RI) greater than 0.5, and a postsystolic notch (⇩) **(Fig. 72.1)**.

RI values of 0.4 - 0.5 in the uterine artery and endometrial vessels may reflect a normal perfusion increase during the second half of the cycle, or they may signify a uterine or endometrial neoplasm **(Table 72.4)**. RI < 0.4 is suspicious for malignancy [6.5].

Uterine myomas **(29)** typically show a peripheral accentuation of vascularity **(Fig. 72.2a)**. The perfusion of myomas decreases in response to hormonal therapy with GnRH analogs, and CDS can be used in these cases to monitor therapeutic response.

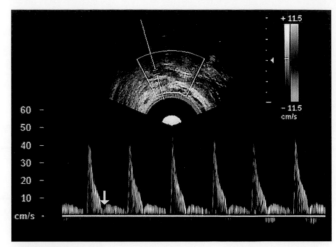

Fig. 72.1

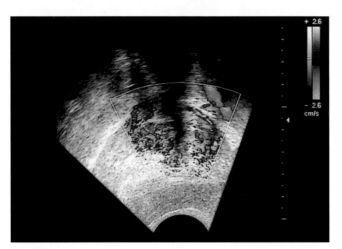

Fig. 72.2a

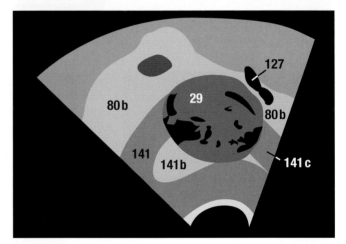

Fig. 72.2b

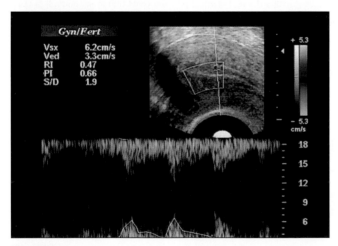

Fig. 72.3a

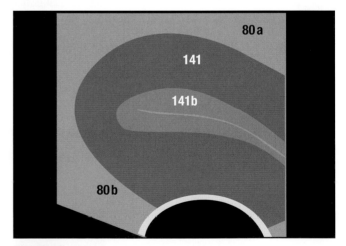

Fig. 72.3b

Hormonal therapy in the setting of in vitro fertilization (IVF) can significantly improve uterine perfusion **(Fig. 72.3a)**. Several studies [6.6] have shown that a PI > 3.0 is associated with suboptimal uterine perfusion and unsuccessful implantation following embryo transfer.

Normal RI values in the uterine artery	
Normal	> 0.50
Borderline	0.50 - 0.40
Suspicious	< 0.40

Table 72.4

Fallopian tubes

Ectopic pregnancy

The incidence of ectopic pregnancy has increased in recent years. Ectopic pregnancy should be suspected when the ß-hCG level is > 6500mlU in a patient with an empty uterine cavity [6.11]. Approximately 96% of all ectopic pregnancies occur in the fallopian tubes, usually the ampullary region. CDS has an adjunctive role in the diagnosis of ectopic pregnancy, since fetal heart activity can be detected in only 10% of ectopic pregnancies **(Fig. 73.1a)** [6.12]. If ectopic pregnancy is suspected on clinical grounds and the adnexal findings are equivocal, ultrasound may demonstrate a typical echogenic ring-like structure in addition to chorionic vascularization **(Fig. 73.1)**.

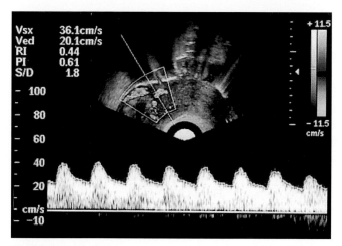

Fig. 73.1a

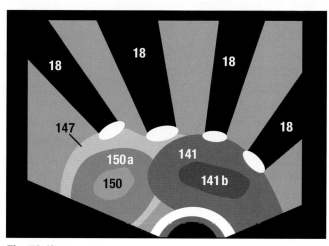

Fig. 73.1b

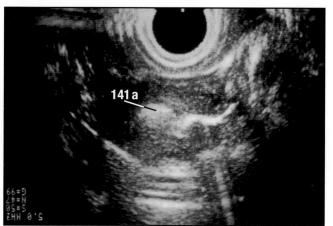

Fig. 73.2

Infertility

Tubal factors are responsible for one-third of female infertility cases. CDS with ultrasound contrast agents can significantly reduce both the costs and risks of infertility evaluations (see p. 107). For transvaginal ultrasound hysterosalpingography, the echogenic agent Echovist® 200 is instilled into the uterine cavity through a transcervical catheter following the exclusion of pelvic inflammatory disease and galactosemia.

B-mode imaging is then performed to define the internal configuration of the uterine cavity **(141a) (Fig. 73.2)** and exclude any anomalies (subseptate or arcuate uterus, etc.). Submucous intracavitary myomas and polyps can also be visualized. Meanwhile the instilled contrast material passes through the cornual, isthmic, and ampullary portions of the fallopian tubes. If the tubes are patent and intact, the contrast material spills into the peritoneum and collects in the cul-de-sac. If sactosalpinx is present, the material will fill the dilated tube without reaching the cul-de-sac.

If a tube is obstructed at the isthmic level, the contrast material will not enter the tube at all. If contrast spillage from the distal end of the tube is questionable, CDS can help by detecting the motion of the flow. This method has a sensitivity of approximately 90% [6.13] and can help to eliminate the need for invasive laparoscopy.

Critical evaluation

CDS is an established noninvasive modality for the surveillance and clinical management of high-risk pregnancies. Numerous randomized studies have documented its diagnostic and clinical value. CDS gives an accurate portrayal of physiologic and pathologic changes in the fetoplacental circulation and provides an important supplement to other surveillance methods (CTG, biophysical profile) that aids in clinical decision-making. Therapeutic decisions, however, should always be made in conjunction with the overall clinical situation and other studies.

In contrast to obstetrics, the use of CDS in the diagnosis of gynecologic masses is still controversial. The lesser pelvis contains numerous vascular systems that have a variety of flow velocities and are subject to cyclical hormonal influences. Moreover, the lack of precise guidelines for performing Doppler measurements places very high demands on the individual responsibility of the examiner.

Training, experience, and a familiarity with CDS are essential for the correct interpretation of suspicious gynecologic findings. It may be necessary to add MRI or CT to the noninvasive workup. After the available findings have been analyzed, a definitive diagnosis should be established by laparoscopy or laparotomy.

Other adjuncts to B-mode imaging are three-dimensional (3-D) ultrasound and 3-D CDS. A three-dimensional rendering can yield additional information based on spatial relationships, volumetric data, and sectional image analysis. 3-D ultrasound can also be used effectively, though infrequently, in the antenatal detection of fetal anomalies - e.g., the exclusion of cleft lip and palate **(Fig. 74.1)**, spina bifida, intracranial masses, vascular malformations, etc. - and in tumor studies, where accurate preoperative planning is required.

A new method in fetal echocardiography, known as cardiac tissue Doppler (CTD), permits color-flow imaging of the cardiac muscle tissue **(Fig. 74.2)**. Prospective clinical studies must still determine whether CTD is superior to conventional color-flow echocardiography or can be a helpful adjunct in the diagnosis of fetal heart disease.

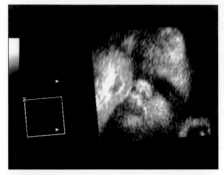

Fig. 74.1

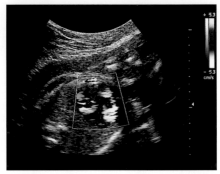

Fig. 74.2

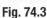

Quiz – Take the following quiz to test your knowledge:

1. When is a Doppler examination indicated during pregnancy? Name at least five different indications.
2. What is meant by the term "cerebroplacental ratio" (CPR)?
3. A 40-year-old woman presents with leukocytosis (WBC 20000) and a suspected left ovarian mass. Her last menstrual period was 3 weeks ago. What criteria would you use to determine whether the mass **(Fig. 74.3)** is benign or malignant? What would you include in the differential diagnosis?
4. A 30-year-old woman presents in her 30th week of pregnancy with IUGR of 4 weeks, abnormal flow in the umbilical artery **(Fig. 74.4)**, and bilateral notching in the placental vessels. Besides the Doppler spectrum, note also the amount of amniotic fluid. What additional studies would you recommended? What would you advise the patient?

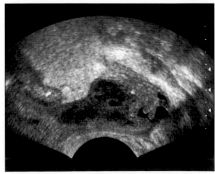

Fig. 74.3 **Fig. 74.4**

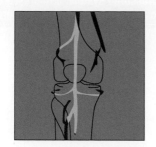

Matthias Hofer

Introduction

A basic diagnostic workup of the peripheral extremity arteries is based on a clinical examination that includes the Ratschow or Allen test, pulse evaluation, walking distance, and measurement of the ankle-brachial index (ABI). Based on these findings, the decision is made whether to proceed with color duplex scanning (CDS) of the extremity.

Intra-arterial digital subtraction angiography (DSA) has been the traditional gold standard in the diagnosis of peripheral arterial occlusive disease (PAOD). But CDS of the peripheral arteries is becoming increasingly important as a noninvasive technique in routine diagnostic situations.

The principal indications for CDS, besides evaluating PAOD and dilatative atherosclerosis, are the quantification of stenosis in PAOD, functional studies, and postoperative follow-up after vascular reconstruction (bypass, endarterectomy, hemodialysis fistula). In a growing number of cases, CDS can eliminate the need for diagnostic DSA prior to interventional and vascular surgical procedures. The compression therapy of false aneurysms (see p. 79) is among the therapeutic applications of CDS, which can help reduce the need for vascular surgical procedures.

Equipment requirements for peripheral arterial CDS include a 3.5-MHz transducer for the pelvic level and a 5-MHz or 7.5-MHz transducer for the distal vessels of the upper and lower extremity, depending on the acoustic conditions (thin or obese patient). Ideally, the patient should rest comfortably in a flat supine position for 15 min before examination of the pelvic, femoral or upper extremity vessels to reduce extraneous influences on blood flow and ensure reproducible results. For examination of the popliteal region or lower leg, the patient should be moved to a lateral decubitus position or, preferably, the prone position. The room temperature should be kept at about 21°C to avoid cold-induced vasoconstriction.

Peripheral Doppler pressure measurements

It is best to use a pocket-size unidirectional CW Doppler probe operating at 8 MHz or 4 MHz. First, measure the brachial systolic pressures on both sides with a Riva-Rocci cuff. Then determine the ankle pressures on each side with the Doppler probe. (A BP cuff is placed about 10cm above the malleolus while the Doppler measurements are performed.) Next, place the Doppler probe behind the malleolus to locate the posterior tibial artery **(87b)**; locate also the dorsal pedal artery **(89a)** and measure the pressures at a beam-vessel angle of approximately 60°. Avoid placing any pressure on the probe. If the pressures are abnormal or if no pressures can be found, locate the peroneal artery **(88a)**. Often it is the best-preserved vessel and can still maintain an adequate blood supply to the lower leg.

Indices: After measuring the systolic pressures, compare the highest ankle pressure to the highest brachial pressure on each side to determine the ankle-brachial index (ABI) and the arm-ankle pressure gradient (AAPG) **(Table 76.1)**. Avoid the sources of over- and underestimation of pressures listed in **Table 76.2**. If a discrepancy is noted between the measured values and clinical complaints, repeat the ABI determination after exercise. A discrepancy of more than 20mmHg in the brachial pressures also warrants further investigation.

A change of >0.15 in the ABI or ≥20mmHg in the AAPG during follow-up suggests a significant increase in vessel narrowing and should be investigated by CDS. A fall in the ankle pressure below 50mmHg is considered critical (risk of necrosis).

| ABI | = | ankle pressure / systolic arm pressure |
| AAPG | = | systolic arm pressure - ankle pressure |

ABI	AAPG	Interpretation
> 1.2	< -20 mmHg	Suspicion of Mönckeberg sclerosis (reducing the compressibility of the vessels)
≥ 0,97	between 0 and -20 mmHg	Normal
0,7 - 0,97	between +5 and + 20 mmHg	Vascular stenosis or well-collateralized occulusions, suspicion of PAOD
< 0,69	> 20 mmHg	Suspicion of poorly collateralized occlusions and multilevel occlusions

Table 76.1

Sources of error in Doppler pressure measurements	
Overestimation of pressures	**Underestimation of pressures**
Positioning the upper body too high	Deflating the cuff too rapidly
Chronic venous insufficiency	Excessive probe pressure
Ankle edema	Insufficient rest period
Hypertension	Hypertension of the ankle joint
Mönckeberg sclerosis	Stenosis between the cuff and probe

Table 76.2

Examination technique in the lower extremity

The examination always starts at the pelvic level. A few selected samplings are sufficient to differentiate physiologic from pathologic findings without having to survey the entire leg.

Initial sampling is limited to the external iliac artery **(84a)**, common femoral artery **(85)**, superficial femoral artery **(85a)**, profunda femoris artery **(85b)**, popliteal artery **(86a)** and, in the lower leg, the anterior tibial artery **(87a)**, posterior tibial artery **(87b)**, and also the peroneal artery **(88a)** if desired **(Fig. 76.3a)**. If abnormalities are found, the entire vascular tree should be examined.

An important vascular region is the bifurcation of the common femoral artery **(85)**, as it is a site of predilection for atherosclerotic disease. If scanning demonstrates an occlusion of the superficial femoral artery **(85a)** (most common location of occlusions in the adductor canal), further attention should be given to the profunda femoris **(85b)** owing to its special importance as a collateral pathway for the lower leg arteries. It is occasionally difficult to trace the vessel below the knee because of its small caliber and during its passage through the adductor canal. It is important to analyze the more distal vascular segments at these levels, as they provide information on the status of the more proximal vascular channels **(Table 78.3)**.

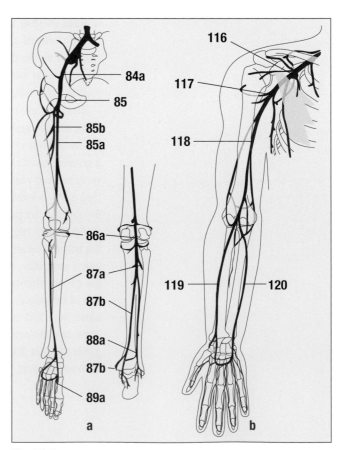

Fig. 76.3

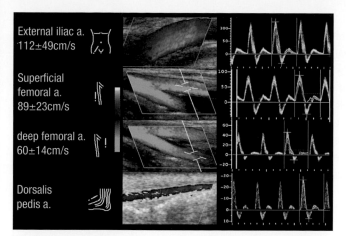

Fig. 77.1

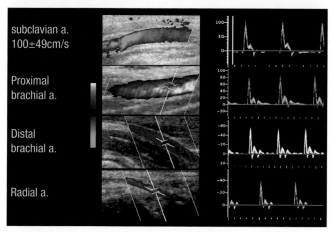

Fig. 77.2

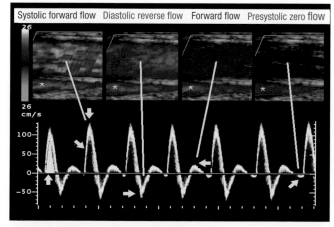

Fig. 77.3 Normal spectrum at rest

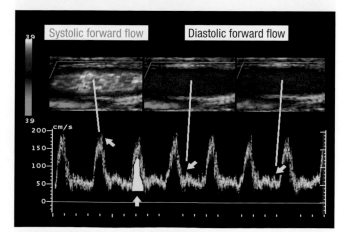

Fig. 77.4 Normal spectrum during exercise

Examination technique in the upper extremity

Examination of the upper extremity always starts at the level of the subclavian artery **(116)** (site of predilection for occlusion), followed by the axillary artery **(117)** and the brachial artery **(118)**. About 1cm distal to the elbow, the brachial artery divides into the radial artery **(119)** and ulnar artery **(120)** **(Fig. 76.3b)**. The proximal and distal portions of both vessels are imaged while the arm is supinated and slightly abducted. Caution: entrapment syndromes may be missed if the arm is not strongly abducted, as this position can suppress typical poststenotic changes in the spectral waveform (see **Table 78.3**).

Normal flow pattern at rest

After identifying the vessels in the B-mode image, examine them with CDS in the longitudinal axis and, if necessary, the transverse axis. Color flow is used initially only in the lower leg and forearm, as it makes it easier to locate and trace the vessels. Adjust the PRF beforehand to the anticipated flow velocity (**Figs. 77.1**, **77.2**; see p.12). For longitudinal scans, use beam steering and carefully adjust the transducer angle to improve the beam-vessel angle and optimize the color-flow image (see p.12). Due to their high peripheral resistance, the spectra from peripheral arteries show a typical triphasic flow pattern **(Fig. 77.3)** consisting of a steep systolic upslope (↘), a systolic peak (↓), a reverse flow component ("dip") in early diastole (⇒), forward flow in late diastole (⇐), and presystolic zero flow (↗). Note the typical continuous flow in the accompanying vein (∗) at each stage of the cardiac cycle.

Normal flow pattern during exercise

Exercise evokes a decrease in peripheral resistance, normally resulting in a biphasic spectrum. This differs from the resting spectrum by the absence of early diastolic reverse flow, a higher level of diastolic flow (↙), and a higher PSV (↖) **(Fig. 77.4)**. Exercise may consist of repetitive fist clenching or circular movements of the foot.

The wall filter should be set to 100 Hz or less, and the sample volume should occupy no more than two-thirds of the vessel lumen to prevent wall artifacts. A clear spectral window (↑) under the systolic peak is a normal finding that signals the absence of slow turbulent flow components. If stenosis is present, the window fills in (see **Fig. 78.4**). The stenosis can be quantified by analyzing the spectral waveform (see **Table 78.3**), determining the peak systolic velocity ratio (PSV ratio, see p.14), or by planimetry in a true cross-sectional image (see **Fig. 81.3b**). A cross-sectional area reduction of at least 30% must be present to produce a detectable spectral change. The PI and RI add little information, as they are subject to large variations due to the varying peripheral resistance (e.g., PI can range from 3 to 30) [7.1]. The flow velocities also vary, of course, but peak systolic velocities should be approximately 100cm/s in the upper leg and approximately 50cm/s in the lower leg **(Figs. 77.1)** [7.6].

Peripheral arterial occlusive disease (PAOD)

Atherosclerosis-related PAOD is the most common disease of the extremity arteries (95%). Color duplex can be used for screening patients with clinically suspected PAOD and for follow-up after surgical treatment. The clinical staging system is summarized in **Table 78.1**. Approximately 10% of the population have peripheral circulatory disease, with 10% of cases involving the upper extremity arteries and 90% the lower extremity arteries (35% pelvis, 50% thigh). Multi-level disease and bilateral involvement are common. The earliest ultrasound sign of incipient atherosclerosis is thickening of the intima and media. Occlusive disease is also manifested by wall changes in the B-mode image (luminal narrowing, soft or hard plaque) and by turbulence and flow irregularities in the color-flow image. The primary tools for the quantification of stenosis are spectral analysis **(Table 78.3)** and determination of the PSV ratio (see p.14).

Figure 78.4 shows an approximately 90% stenosis of the common femoral artery with typical intra- and poststenotic spectral changes. Note that the prestenotic PSV may be markedly reduced in the presence of multilevel disease, and therefore the relative PSV increase is used as a criterion for stenosis. When a transverse image is available, the original and residual luminal areas can be determined by planimetric analysis (see **Fig.81.3b**). When a thrombotic occlusion is found, the length of the occluded segment should be determined. Slow blood flow or shadowing plaque in the more distal vascular segment can cause the length of the occlusion to be underestimated.

Staging of chronic PAOD (Fontaine classification)	
Stage I:	Stenoses or occlusions with no clinical symptoms
Stage II a:	Intermittent claudication with walking distance > 200 m
II b:	Intermittent claudication with walking distance < 200 m
Stage III:	Rest pain
Stage IV a:	Ischemia with trophic disturbances and necrosis
IV b:	Ischemia with moist gangrene

Table 78.1

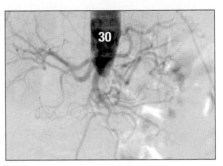

Fig. 78.2

Leriche Syndrome

A special form of PAOD is the Leriche syndrome, which refers to chronic thrombosis (⤴) of the aortic bifurcation **(30)** with bilateral absence of the common femoral artery pulses. An extensive collateral circulation (⇒) **(Figs. 78.2, 78.5)** generally develops to compensate for the occlusion, which is often detected incidentally in patients evaluated for intermittent claudication of the hip or for erectile dysfunction (see p.56). Note how the decreased peripheral resistance produces a biphasic waveform in the inferior epigastric artery (⇒ , **Fig.78.5**), which functions as a collateral channel.

Criteria for stenosis in spectral analysis				
Percent stenosis	Prestenotic spectrum	Intrastenotic spectrum	Spectrum just past the stenosis	Spectrum far distal to the stenosis
0–50%	Normal: – Triphasic or biphasic – Narrow frequency band – Clear spectral window	– Increase in PSV (by <100% and/or <180 cm/s)	– No significant turbulence – Possible flow reversal	– Same as prestenotic
51–75%	Normal	– Increase in PSV (>100% and/or >180 cm/s) – Slight decrease in pulsatility	– Flow reversal – Possible slight turbulence – Some fill-in of spectral window	– Pulsatility normal or slightly reduced
76–99%	– Normal or slightly reduced velocity – Pulsatility increased	– Increase in PSV (>250% and/or >180 cm/s) – Pulsatility decreased	– Significant turbulence – Complete fill-in of spectral window	– Reduced PSV – Reduced pulsatility – Flattened systolic peak
100%	– Low velocity – Increased pulsatility – Narrow complex with high reverse flow component	– No flow signal	– Slight flow in distal connecting vessel due to collaterals	– Very flat systolic peak

Table 78.3

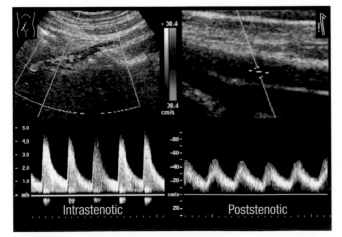

Fig. 78.4

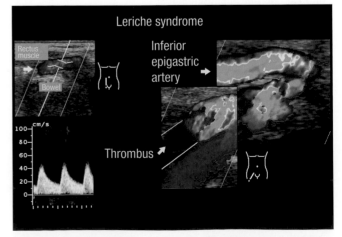

Fig. 78.5 Documentation of collateral flow in Leriche syndrome

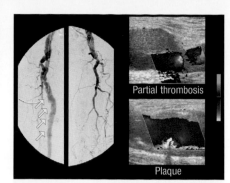

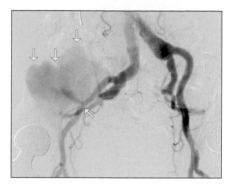

Partial thrombosis

Plaque

Fig. 79.1

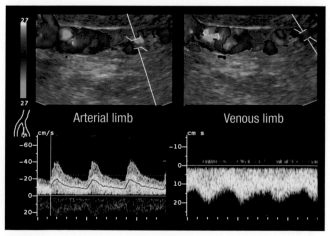

Arterial limb

Venous limb

Fig. 79.2

True aneurysm, false aneurysm, dissecting aneurysm

The key points in aneurysm diagnosis are to determine the precise extent of the aneurysm, evaluate the perfused lumen (thrombi are a potential embolism source), and identify dissection of the vessel wall. A true aneurysm is a dilatation that encompasses all the layers of the vessel wall (see p.35). This lesion frequently affects the popliteal artery and may be solitary or multifocal **(Fig. 79.1** ↗).

False aneurysms **(Fig. 79.2** ⇩ **)** most commonly result from iatrogenic arterial puncture, in this case of the distal external iliac artery (◥). They can also develop at suture sites following vascular surgery. The main complications of false aneurysm are rupture and adjacent nerve compression. The aneurysmal mass consists of a perivascular hematoma that communicates with the vessel lumen. CDS typically shows uniform bidirectional flow in the aneurysm neck **(Fig. 79.3a)**. Therapeutically, the operator can induce thrombosis of the perfused hematoma by applying compression under CDS guidance **(Fig. 79.3b)** [7.4]. Contraindications are aneurysms above the inguinal ligament, an aneurysm more than 7cm in diameter, and preexisting ischemia of the extremity. Similar results can be achieved by vascular compression with a pneumatic device (FemoStop) [7.8]. The rate of spontaneous pseudoaneurysm thrombosis is only about 30-58% [7.4].

Arteriovenous malformation (AVM)

AVMs may be congenital or acquired as a result of puncture (AV fistula) or vascular trauma (in approximately 0.7% of cardiac catheterizations [7.3]). An AVM is an abnormal communication between the high-pressure arterial system and low-pressure venous system. This produces typical flow disturbances and spectral changes both proximal and distal to the fistula and in its venous limb. With the decreased peripheral resistance on the venous side, the spectrum is biphasic proximal to the fistula **(Fig. 79.4)** and triphasic distal to the fistula. Arterial inflow into the venous limb causes turbulence and arterial pulsations, which can also be visualized **(Fig. 79.4)**. A large shunt volume places a potentially harmful volume load on the heart (see p. 81).

Arterial compression syndromes

Arterial compression syndromes result from the persistent or recurrent (e.g., due to postural changes) constriction of neurovascular structures due to various causes, leading to deficient perfusion of the more distal vascular tree. The unphysiologic stresses on the compressed vascular segment lead to intimal lesions that predispose to stenosis, thrombosis, and embolism. The major compression syndromes of the upper extremity are the thoracic outlet and thoracic inlet syndromes. The most common manifestation in the lower extremity is the popliteal entrapment syndrome. Contraction of the calf muscles alters the relationship between the popliteal artery and medial gastrocnemius muscle, causing compression of the artery. This is causative in approximately 40% of intermittent claudication cases occurring before age 30. CDS can demonstrate the change in flow pattern during exercise and the anatomic interrelationship of the vessels and muscles.

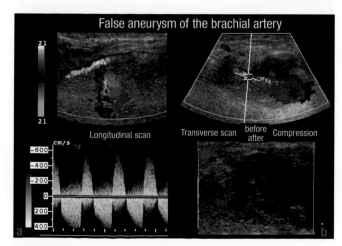

False aneurysm of the brachial artery

Longitudinal scan   Transverse scan   before/after   Compression

Fig. 79.3

Fig. 79.4

Follow-up after bypass insertion

CDS can directly evaluate the success of vascular bypass surgery and can also detect possible complications such as restenosis and bypass occlusion at an early stage. The proximal and distal anastomosis in the bypass itself (✍) should be examined for flow irregularities, and PSV measurements should be obtained at three points **(Fig. 80.3)**. The criteria for bypass stenosis are shown in **Table 80.1**. The echogenic walls (⬎) of vascular prostheses or stents and the acoustic shadow (↗) cast by the stent material should not be misinterpreted as plaque or restenosis.

Vessel-stent junctions and anastomotic suture lines form sites of predilection for restenosis. The most frequent causes are listed in **Table 80.2**.

If the spectrum shows low amplitude, high pulsatility, and a high reverse-flow component, it is very likely that an occlusion is present **(Fig. 80.4)**. An occlusion (↖) of the common femoral artery is manifested by a cutoff of color flow and an absence of spectral flow signals just behind the distal bypass anastomosis (⇓). What is the cause of the different angled shadows (↗) in **Fig. 80.3** ? (See above.)

Follow-up after PTA

Figure 80.5a shows the site where flow is reconstituted distal to an occlusion of the superficial femoral artery. Because of peripheral vasodilatation, flow distal to the occlusion has a typical biphasic spectrum **(Fig. 80.5b)** with a reduced PSV (⇐) and increased late-diastolic flow (⇑). The follow-up examination after successful percutaneous transluminal angioplasty (PTA) shows a marked increase in PSV (⇒) **(Fig. 80.6)** with normal late-diastolic flow (⇓). Fill-in of the spectral window is based on the early postinterventional timing of the examination. There has been insufficient time for smoothing of the intima, resulting in persistence of turbulent flow.

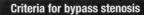

Criteria for bypass stenosis
PSV ≤ 45 cm/s
PSV > 250 cm/s
Change in the PSV ratio of > 2,5 (most reliable parameter for stenoses >50% [7.7])

Table 80.1

Causes of recurrent stenosis
Acute thrombosis
Vascular dissection after PTA due to intimal-medial tears
Improperly dilated stent
Irregularities at the junction of the bypass or stent with the blood vessel
Myointimal hyperplasia
Progression of underlying disease
Infection

Table 80.2

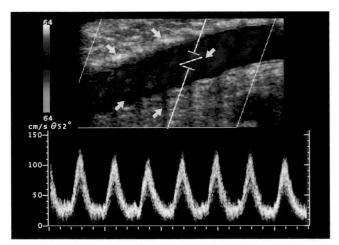

Fig. 80.3

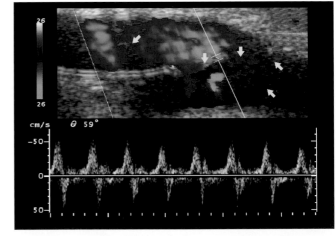

Fig. 80.4

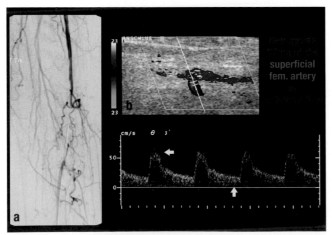

Fig. 80.5

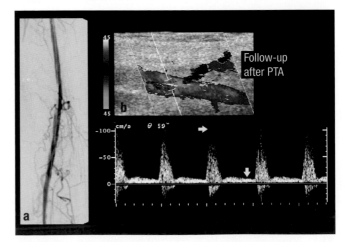

Fig. 80.6

Formula for calculating flow in a hemodialysis fistula

$$Vol = \pi \cdot r^2 \cdot V_{mean} \cdot 60$$

Vol: Volume flow in ml/min

r: Radius (1/2 diameter) in cm

V_{mean}:   Average flow velocity in cm/s (V_{mean} represents the time-averaged velocity, not the average peak velocity.)

Table 81.1

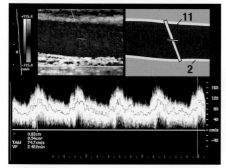

Fig. 81.2

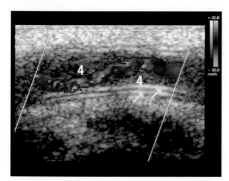

Fig. 81.3 a

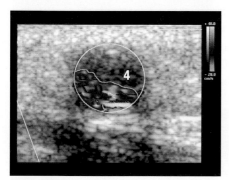

Fig. 81.3 b

Evaluation of hemodialysis fistulas

High-frequency linear-array transducers (e.g., 7.5MHz) are used in the evaluation of AV fistulas for hemodialysis access. Because of the difficulty in assigning CDS findings to anatomic structures, the examination should be performed in consultation with the attending dialysis physician or surgeon. We recommend the following protocol:

1) Always start at the brachial artery when examining the inflow artery, which is usually imaged in transverse section. The spectrum should show a definite low-resistance pattern with strong diastolic flow. If this is not the case, it should be assumed that fistula malfunction is present. A high-resistance pattern means that incoming arterial blood is not flowing freely into the fistula, and that therefore the flow is restricted at some point by stenosis.

2) Several duplex volume flow measurements (at least three, preferably six) should be obtained in the inflow artery. This is best done in the brachial artery several centimeters above the elbow. These measurements are essential both for follow-up and for general evaluation. A volume flow of <300ml/min in a Cimino fistula or <550ml/min in a Gore-Tex graft signifies insufficiency. The respective lower cutoff values for "normal" fistulas are 600 and 800ml/min.

3) The course of the inflow artery is examined for signs of stenosis (flow acceleration and turbulence). There is no velocity cutoff value that can confirm a stenosis. Detection relies on the measurement of cross-sectional area reduction relative to normal prestenotic and poststenotic segments in the B-mode image. This also applies to stenoses in the venous limb of the fistula. The vein should be scanned with a "floating" transducer applied with very little pressure, as any compression will cause major artifacts. The access vein is examined as far as the central veins for signs of stenosis, aneurysm, perivascular hematoma, or partial thrombosis. As in DSA, the quantification of stenoses is hampered by the lack of a reference value given the varying luminal widths in the course of the access vein. The following are typical sites of occurrence for stenosis:
   - The anastomotic area between the artery and draining vein
   - The site where the fistula is usually accessed
   - The central veins (e.g., following central venous catheter placement in the subclavian or internal jugular vein)
   - With a Gore-Tex fistula: the distal anastomosis between the Gore-Tex graft and the draining vein.

Figure 81.2 illustrates the measurement of volume flow in the brachial artery. This artery was scanned at a high angle due to the unfavorable course of the vessel, which ran almost parallel to the transducer face. The sample volume **(11)** spans the full diameter of the artery **(1)**. The blood flow shows a definite low-resistance pattern. With a volume flow of nearly 2.5l/min, the patient's heart failure could be attributed to the increased fistula flow. Heart failure regressed following surgical closure of the fistula after renal transplantation.

Figure 81.3 a shows a long, high-grade segmental stenosis in a Gore-Tex fistula. The Gore-Tex material is recognized by the double contour (⤢⤢) of the fistula wall. Quantification of the stenosis is best performed in transverse section **(Fig. 81.3 b)** by measuring the total vascular area and the perfused, color-filled area in relation to the hypoechoic thrombus **(4)**. Calculation indicates a 75% luminal reduction.

Critical evaluation

The noninvasive modalities of CDS and MRA have been gaining clinical importance owing to their lack of ionizing radiation in frequent follow-ups and their benefits in patients with contrast allergies, renal failure, or autonomous thyroid adenomas.

While DSA is an invasive study that is useful only for topographic mapping, CDS can additionally furnish differential diagnostic information on stenotic lesions, functional parameters, and reactions in surrounding tissues. It can also detect the presence of thrombi in aneurysms. In the hands of an experienced sonographer, CDS is an excellent noninvasive option for the examination of peripheral vessels.

The traditional disadvantages of CDS, such as the limited visualization of vessels that are deeply situated or obscured by calcifications, have been significantly reduced, owing particularly to the use of ultrasound contrast agents. **Figure 82.1b** shows how the administration of a contrast enhancer improved the detection of a tibial artery stenosis that was poorly visualized without contrast medium **(Fig. 82.1a)**.

The SieScape panoramic imaging technique, when combined with power Doppler, can significantly improve the documentation of pathology involving a long vascular segment **(Fig. 82.2)**. The combination of these techniques can provide a topographic survey of vascular changes up to 60cm in length [7.4].

CDS is often of limited value for studies of the lower leg vessels, especially when small calibers, multiple plaques, and slow flow are present due to multilevel disease. DSA is still the modality of choice for evaluating arterial disease below the knee.

Besides CDS, it appears that gadolinium-enhanced MRI and phase-contrast MRA of the peripheral vessels will one day become an attractive alternative to invasive DSA [7.2]. CT angiography, on the other hand, is of no current importance in peripheral vascular studies. Its drawbacks include artifacts from calcium-containing plaques, the need for high doses of intravenous contrast medium, and high radiation exposure from long acquisition times. It is best used for detecting aneurysms in centrally located vessels [7.2].

Evaluation of hemodialysis fistulas

CDS is markedly superior to angiography in several respects. Besides its ability to measure volume flow, CDS can often furnish an etiologic diagnosis, for example, by identifying pressure from a hematoma as the cause of luminal narrowing. CDS is also useful for follow-up examinations. When the volume flow is known, it is easier to evaluate the significance of a stenosis than when angiography is used. Thus, a wait-and-see approach may be taken with a moderate to higher-grade stenosis if the fistula flow is considered satisfactory.

Initial prospective and randomized studies have shown that regular CDS examinations at 6-month intervals, with prophylactic dilatation of stenoses of more than 50%, can significantly prolong hemodialysis access survival and reduce costs [7.9].

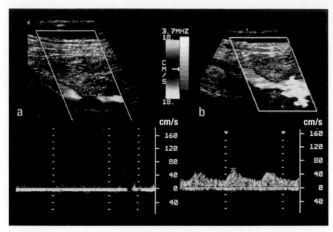

Fig. 82.1

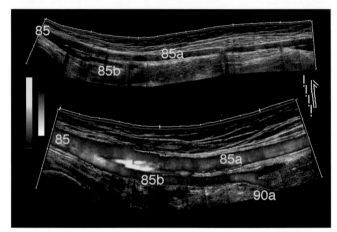

Fig. 82.2

Quiz – Take the following quiz to test your knowledge:

1. **Figure 82.3** shows an approximately 80% stenosis. In the blue squares, draw the spectral waveforms that would correspond to levels **b** and **c** and identify the vessels that are shown. Note that the systolic velocity is already markedly reduced at the prestenotic level (**a**). What accounts for this low PSV?

2. What makes it difficult to determine the length of an arterial thrombosis? (answer on page 78)

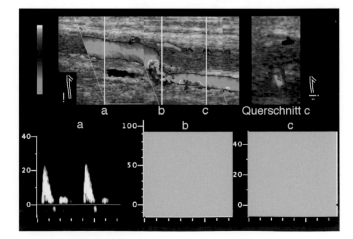

Fig. 82.3

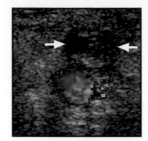

Andreas Saleh

Introduction

The different vascular territories of the upper and lower extremities are characterized by distinctive pathophysiologic phenomena and therefore are discussed under separate headings. The examination technique must conform to the peculiar circumstances of the regional anatomy. Nevertheless, the information presented under a particular heading applies to other headings as well, which is why this chapter on peripheral veins stands as a separate educational unit.

Deep vein thrombosis (DVT) is of primary interest in the deep venous system of the lower extremity. Major risk factors are posttraumatic or postoperative immobilization, long-distance flights or bus travel, paraneoplastic syndromes, and hypercoagulopathies. The clinical signs of DVT are confusing, and doubtful cases are resolved by imaging evaluation, giving particular attention to the DVT checklist shown on the left (Table 83.1).

Most circulatory problems in the superficial venous system of the lower extremity are based on valvular incompetence (venous insufficiency). Primary varicosity is a disease of the superficial lower extremity veins in which the venous valves are unable to close due to causes that are not fully understood. Secondary varicosity results from an increased volume load on the superficial venous system, which functions as a collateral pathway when DVT is present (postthrombotic syndrome). Primary and secondary varicose veins can lead to the clinical picture of chronic venous insufficiency (CVI). Imaging evaluation should focus on the questions listed in Table 83.2.

Thrombosis of the superficial veins (thrombophlebitis) is usually a clinical diagnosis and rarely necessitates imaging studies.

Thrombosis of the upper extremity (Paget-von Schroetter syndrome) is rare. Usually it is a catheter-related complication or results from physical overexertion (effort thrombosis). Clinical manifestations are usually pronounced (arm swelling), and the main purpose of imaging is to confirm the clinical impression.

Checklist for DVT

1. Is thrombosis present?

2. What is the extent of the thrombosis?

3. What is the age of the thrombosis?

4. Is the thrombus adherent to the vessel wall?

5. What is the cause of the thrombosis?

Table 83.1

Checklist for CVI

1. Is venous insufficiency present?

2. What are the proximal and distal limits of the venous insufficiency?

3. Is there an anomalous saphenofemoral or saphenopopliteal termination?

4. Is the deep venous system patent and competent?

Table 83.2

Basic principles in the diagnosis of thrombosis

A healthy vein can be completely compressed with the ultrasound probe **(Fig. 84.1b)**, but it cannot be compressed when filled with thrombotic material **(Fig. 84.1c)**. This compression test is carried out in cross-section because the beam may deviate laterally in longitudinal section and mimic compressibility, resulting in a false-negative diagnosis of thrombosis.

Thrombi cannot be reliably detected in the B-mode image because they are often as hypoechoic as flowing blood. Color flow is initially used only for navigation as it makes vessels easier to locate. With a good B-mode image, the compression test can be carried out without color flow. The decisive criterion is not the ability to "push away the color" but the complete compressibility of the vessel lumen. With a poor B-mode image, it is better to activate color flow and combine it with distal compression (↰) if necessary. The most elegant technique is to combine both aspects with a rocking hand motion: To do this, first apply distal pressure with the hypothenar eminence of the hand holding the probe **(Fig. 84.2a)**. Identify the vein (at least partially patent) by the resulting flow acceleration, and immediately apply probe compression (↓ in **Fig. 84.2b**). **Figure 84.3** illustrates this "see-saw test" carried out on the peroneal group of veins. Spontaneous flow signals are not detected initially in the peroneal veins (↑ in **Fig. 84.3a**). When distal compression is applied **(Fig. 84.2a)**, flow acceleration (↗) can be seen **(Fig. 84.3b)**. Second, completely compress the vein with the probe **(Fig. 84.2b**, ⇐ in **Fig. 84.3c)**. Note that only the vein segment that is compressed can be evaluated. Thus it is necessary to scan all the leg veins over their entire course while applying intermittent compression. Since this requires an experienced examiner, who is not always available, algorithms have been developed that can limit the compression test to two points on the lower extremity: the groin and the popliteal fossa. When this is combined with a blood test (D-dimers), thrombosis can be diagnosed with a reasonably high degree of confidence [8.1].

Practical anatomy

The deep veins of the lower extremity accompany the homonymous arteries. The veins are generally paired in the lower leg. To define the anterior tibial veins **(130a)**, the probe is placed on the tibialis anterior muscle **(139)**, which is easily identified by palpation lateral to the anterior tibial margin **(Fig. 84.4a)**. The anterior group of lower leg veins runs posterior to the extensor muscles and just anterior to the interosseous membrane **(134)**. The beginner usually scans too deeply when attempting to locate these veins. The interosseous margins of the tibia **(21f)** and fibula **(21e)** mark the level of the interosseous membrane, which can be directly visualized **(134)**.

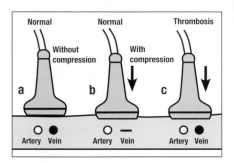

Fig. 84.1

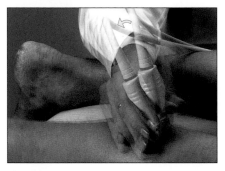

Fig. 84.2a

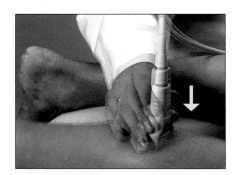

Fig. 84.2b

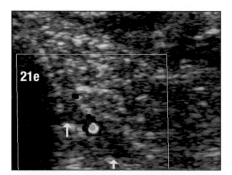

Fig. 84.3a

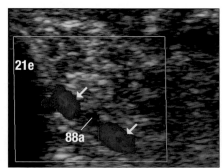

Fig. 84.3b

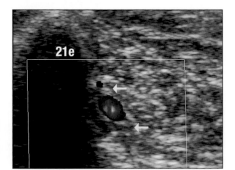

Fig. 84.3c

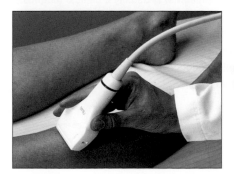

Fig. 84.4a

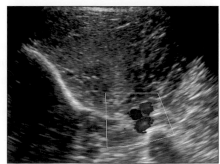

Fig. 84.4b

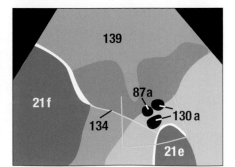

Fig. 84.4c

The posterior tibial veins **(130b)** and peroneal veins **(88b)** are located in the flexor compartment between the triceps surae muscle **(132)** and the deep flexors **(133)**. Bony landmarks are used for orientation: when the leg is held in the neutral position, the posterior tibial surface **(21f)** is more anterior than the posterior fibular surface **(21e)**. The posterior tibial veins **(130b)** are approximately centered over the posterior tibial surface, while the peroneal veins **(88b)** are in very close proximity to the fibula **(Fig. 85.1)**.

The landmark for identifying the popliteal vein **(86b)** is the accompanying artery **(86a)**, which runs anterior to the vein. The vein is easy to find owing to its large caliber and superficial location **(Fig. 85.2)**. Even slight transducer pressure is often sufficient to compress the vein completely, causing it to disappear from the image. The popliteal vein is paired in approximately 20% of cases and triple in approximately 2%. The femoral vein lies posterior to the artery in the adductor canal, becoming medial to the artery at a more proximal level. The iliac vein runs posteromedial to the accompanying artery. The deep femoral vein enters the superficial femoral vein 4-12cm below the inguinal ligament. It runs anterior to the homonymous artery. The superficial femoral vein is paired in approximately 20% of cases, and three or more veins exist in 14% of cases.

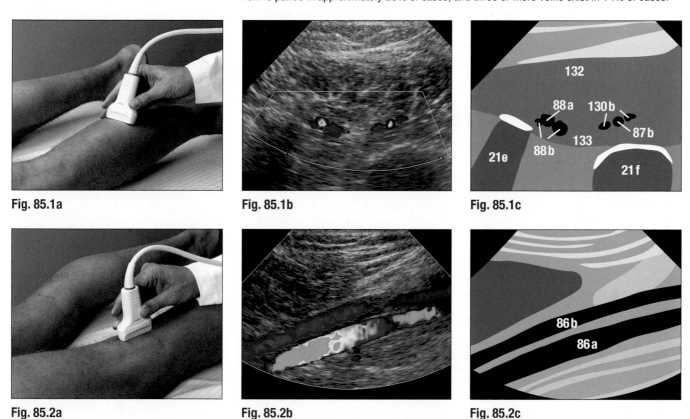

Fig. 85.1a   Fig. 85.1b   Fig. 85.1c

Fig. 85.2a   Fig. 85.2b   Fig. 85.2c

Examination technique

For duplex examination of the lower extremity, the patient is positioned supine with the upper body slightly elevated. Start the examination at the groin using a 4-7MHz linear-array transducer. Trace the femoral vein distally to the femoral epicondyle while applying intermittent compression. Note also the course of the deep femoral vein. Continue down the leg and scan the anterior tibial veins before moving the patient to the prone position. A small cushion is placed below the ankle to flex the knee slightly. Visualize the popliteal vein in transverse section. First trace the vessel proximally while applying intermittent compression (often the distal adductor canal is visualized better from a posterior than anterior approach). Next trace the vessel distally and separately evaluate the posterior peroneal and tibial groups of veins. Be careful when examining the proximal peroneal veins. Because of the physiologic ectasia of the peroneal veins and the normal skin tension over the fibular head, strong and often painful pressure must be exerted to compress these veins. The conclusion of the examination depends on the findings to this point and on the clinical context **(Table 86.6)**. Conclude either by examining the common femoral vein while the patient performs a Valsalva maneuver or by color-flow imaging of the iliac veins using a 4-7MHz convex transducer array.

If you cannot adequately evaluate the lower leg veins using this standard protocol, try flexing the knee over the edge of the bed or table while the leg is relaxed. Cradle the lower leg in the left hand while scanning with the right hand. The increased hydrostatic pressure results in better filling of the veins, which makes them easier to identify. On the negative side, color flow imaging is less rewarding because of the slow blood flow, and considerably more transducer pressure is needed to compress the veins than in the recumbent position.

Pathologic findings

An abnormal compression test confirms the presence of thrombosis. An incomplete thrombosis (↖) is partially compressible (see **Fig. 86.4**). Extent is determined by locating the proximal end of the thrombus and documenting it with longitudinal and transverse scans. Accurate documentation of the anatomic location of the proximal end is crucial for follow-up. The proximal end of a fresh thrombus is usually nonadherent to the vessel wall, although the term "free floating thrombus" should be avoided as it is ambiguous and its clinical relevance is unclear. The best way to estimate the age of thrombosis is to determine the diameter of the thrombosed vein in relation to the accompanying artery. The transverse diameter of a fresh thrombus (⇒⇐) (<10 days old) in the lower extremity is more than twice the diameter of the accompanying artery **(A)** **(Fig. 86.1)**. Older thrombi (⇒⇐) have a smaller diameter due to clot retraction **(Fig. 86.2)**. The measurement is documented with images. The echogenicity of a thrombus is not a reliable indicator of its age.

The standard protocol in patients with suspected DVT is to examine not just the lower extremity veins but the entire leg and pelvis. Occasionally this will disclose the cause of the DVT, such as a pelvic mass leading to flow obstruction. Even small lesions, such as the isolated thrombosis of a muscle vein **(131)**, can cause severe pain **(Fig. 86.3)**. Baker cysts **(110)** are particularly common in patients with rheumatoid arthritis. **Figure 86.5** illustrates a Baker cyst, the neck of which (✍) communicates with the posterior joint space of the knee.

Specific problems and solutions

Poor visualization of the femoral vein in the adductor canal.
Support the thigh from behind with the left hand during the examination. Otherwise try a posterior approach for imaging the distal portions of the adductor canal.

The leg appears too swollen for ultrasound examination.
First consider alternative modalities. If this is not possible, locate the femoral vein in the groin and also locate the popliteal vein. Both sites can always be evaluated with ultrasound. The findings, though minimal, are useful for selecting therapeutic options when thrombosis is present.

Thrombosis is present, but the pelvic vessels are difficult to evaluate.
The external iliac vein can almost always be evaluated in its distal portion, but often the proximal end of the thrombus cannot be seen. There is usually no difficulty in compressing the vena cava, however. This finding is usually adequate if conservative treatment is desired, since ultrasound has demonstrated involvement at the pelvic level while excluding vena cava thrombosis.

Thrombosis is absent, but the pelvic vessels are difficult to evaluate.
If there is no reason to suspect that isolated pelvic vein thrombosis is present (e.g., pelvic mass, malignant lymphoma), thrombosis at that level can be indirectly excluded by a normal response of the common femoral vein to a Valsalva maneuver.

Significant atherosclerosis of the accompanying arteries creates acoustic shadows that obscure the veins.
Try changing the transducer position to scan past the artery and interrogate the vein directly.

The veins in the lower leg cannot be positively identified.
In a patient with a very thick calf, adjust the transducer position to minimize the distance from the transducer face to the veins of interest. If they still cannot be adequately visualized, try flexing the leg over the edge of the table (see above).

Table 86.6

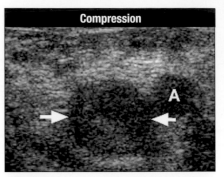

Fig. 86.1

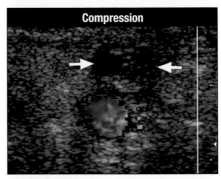

Fig. 86.2

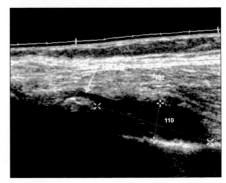

Fig. 86.3

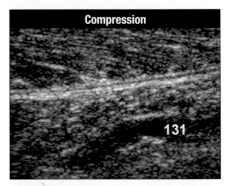

Fig. 86.5

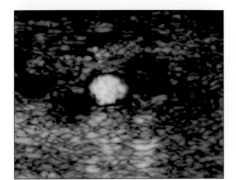

Fig. 86.4 a

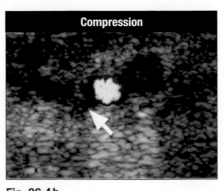

Fig. 86.4 b

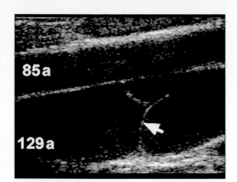

Fig. 87.1

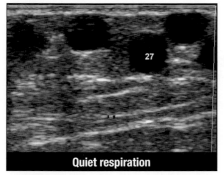

Quiet respiration

Fig. 87.2a

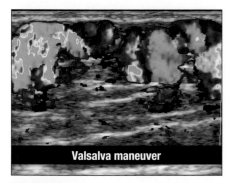

Valsalva maneuver

Fig. 87.2b

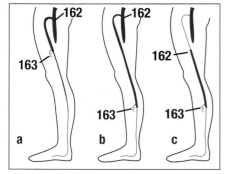

Fig. 87.3

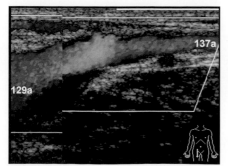

Fig. 87.4a

Venous insufficiency examination

Although venous valves (🖎) can be directly visualized with ultrasound under favorable conditions **(Fig. 87.1)**, the diagnosis of venous insufficiency is based on indirect criteria. While the proximal pressure is increased by having the patient perform a Valsalva maneuver or by applying proximal manual compression (see p. 84), the examiner attempts to record a distal reflux signal **(Fig. 87.2b)** that competent venous valves would have prevented. Complete saphenous varicosity starts with incompetence at the level of the terminal valve and, with passage of time, progresses to more distal levels. As a result, the blood that fills the (incompetent) superficial vein comes from the deep venous system. When the proximal pressure is increased (e.g., by a Valsalva maneuver), the deep venous valves will close if the deep venous system is competent, allowing reflux to occur only between the terminal valve of the superficial vein and the next most proximal deep venous valve. This segment is quite large in the case of the great saphenous vein, but the popliteal vein contains so many valves that the reflux volume is small. As a result, it is more difficult to detect small saphenous varicosity than great saphenous varicosity.

The most proximal incompetent venous valve marks the proximal reflux point **(162)**, or the proximal limit of the venous insufficiency. The first competent valve in the varicose vein marks the distal reflux point **(163)**. The proximal and distal reflux points provide a basis for the classification of saphenous varicosity **(Fig. 87.3)**. The proximal reflux point usually consists of an incompetent saphenofemoral valve (complete saphenous varicosity, **Fig. 87.3a, b)**. The level of the distal reflux point determines the severity (anatomic extent) of the varicosity in the Hach classification: grade I, proximal thigh; grade II, distal thigh **(Fig. 87.3a)**; grade III, proximal lower leg **(Fig. 87.3b)**; grade IV, distal lower leg. A similar three-grade classification is used for the small saphenous vein. If the proximal reflux point is located distal to the terminal valve, the saphenous varicosity is classified as incomplete **(Fig. 87.3c)**.

Practical anatomy

The great saphenous vein **(137a)** starts at the medial border of the foot, runs anterior to the medial malleolus, and enters the femoral vein approximately 3cm below the inguinal ligament **(Fig. 87.3)**. There are variants in which the great saphenous vein terminates in the superficial epigastric vein (anomalous proximal termination) or in the femoral vein below the venous confluence (anomalous distal termination).

The small saphenous vein **(137b)** starts at the lateral border of the foot, ascends behind the lateral malleolus, and enters the popliteal vein 3-8cm above the joint line of the knee. The terminal portion of the small saphenous vein is subfascial and inaccessible to inspection. Normally the long and small saphenous veins taper toward the periphery (telescope sign, **Fig. 87.4a)**. A tubular, nontapered vessel with forward flow is a sign of extrafascial collateralization in deep vein thrombosis **(Fig. 87.4b)**, while a tubular vessel with reversed flow indicates venous insufficiency. The marked decrease of flow velocity in incompetent veins **(27)** can produce spontaneous intraluminal echoes (🖎) **(Fig. 87.5)**. These echoes disappear at once when transducer pressure is applied.

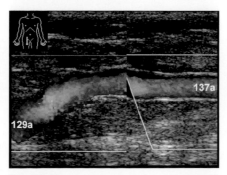

Fig. 87.4b

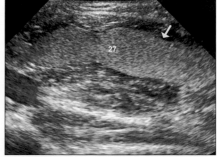

Fig. 87.5

Examination technique and findings

The patient is examined in a standing position with the leg relaxed. Alternatively, the leg may be flexed over a table edge for examining varicose veins below the knee. After the terminal portions of the saphenous veins have been identified, the proximal pressure is increased to test the function of the terminal valves. The test is repeated at various levels to locate the distal limit of the venous insufficiency. The vein is compressed proximally during a Valsalva maneuver to determine whether pure saphenous insufficiency is present or whether there are additional tributaries (incompetent side branches, perforator incompetence). In this way the proximal limit of the venous insufficiency can be determined in patients with incomplete saphenous varicosity. Incompetent perforating veins can be directly visualized with CDS. There is no need for a tourniquet like that used in CW Doppler. It is impractical to scan the entire lower extremity for incompetent perforating veins, and the examination should be limited to clinically suspicious areas (e.g., blowouts, typical skin changes).

Thrombosis examination in the upper extremity

Upper extremity thrombosis most commonly affects the subclavian vein. Because this vein is located behind the clavicle, the compression test cannot be used. It is also difficult to compress the proximal and middle thirds of the axillary vein. Thus, the major criterion for diagnosing upper extremity thrombosis is the detection of a color flow void. Color artifacts can be misleading, of course. **Figure 88.2a** shows a partial thrombosis that is difficult to detect (↗) because of excessive color gain. When compression is applied **(Fig. 88.2b)** and when the vessel is scanned in longitudinal section at proper sensitivity **(Fig. 88.2c)**, the true extent of the thrombosis (↙) can be appreciated. Other important veins in the shoulder, neck, and arm can be scanned and compressed as described above (see p. 84). The examination can be supplemented by the use of provocative maneuvers as in the lower extremity, and distal compression is used in the same way. The upper extremity differs from the leg in that deep inspiration tends to accelerate venous flow by lowering the intrathoracic pressure.

Findings and pitfalls

Echogenic lumen (suspected thrombosis)

Intravascular echoes can be caused by overamplification of the B-mode image (B-mode gain too high) or unfavorable acoustic conditions.

Echo-free lumen (no sign of thrombosis)

Fresh thrombi may appear sonolucent (see **Fig. 89.2**).

No detectable flow signal in the vessel lumen (suspected thrombosis)

Very slow flow may be below the threshold of detection even with optimum instrument settings (see p. 16). Often a color signal cannot be obtained just proximal or distal to thrombosis, in the lower leg, or in a standing examination. Shadowing from calcified plaque in the accompanying artery can prevent color flow imaging.

Detectable flow signal in the vessel lumen (no sign of thrombosis)

Thrombosis that is incomplete or partially recanalized may produce a detectable flow signal, so make certain that color fills the lumen before excluding thrombosis. Occasionally this is difficult to achieve even in healthy subjects, which is why distal compression is often used. This technique may cause a partial thrombosis to become swamped with echoes, however **(Fig. 88.2a)**.

Table 88.1

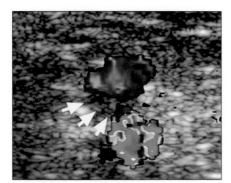

Fig. 88.2a

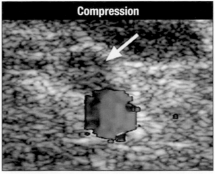

Fig. 88.2b

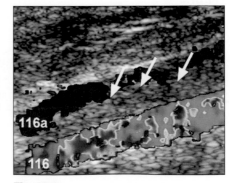

Fig. 88.2c

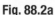

Practical anatomy

Examination of the upper extremity veins is complicated by the "hidden" position of the subclavian vein behind the clavicle **(21c)**. The supraclavicular portion of the vein **(116a) (Fig. 89.1c)** is anterior to the subclavian artery **(116)**. Since the transducer is angled toward the clavicle, usually the vein can only be imaged in longitudinal section. At the infraclavicular level, the transducer is placed in a perpendicular position with its upper edge touching the clavicle **(Fig. 89.1a)**. It is moved along the bone to visualize the subclavian vessels at the junction of the medial and middle thirds of the clavicle. The vein runs anterior to the artery and merges with the axillary vein **(117a)** at the lateral margin of the first rib. The brachial veins and the antebrachial veins have narrow calibers and are of minor clinical importance.

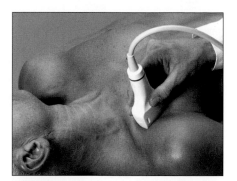

Fig. 89.1a

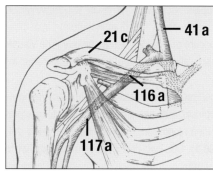

Fig. 89.1b

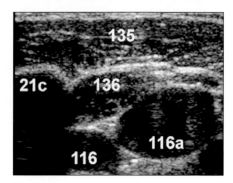

Fig. 89.1c

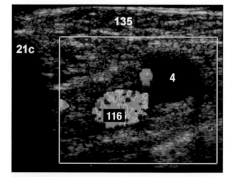

Fig. 89.2

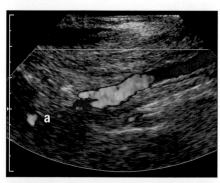

Fig. 89.3

Examination technique and findings

For examination of the upper extremity, position the patient supine with the upper body slightly elevated. Place the patient's arm on your lap and adjusts its position as needed with your left hand. Start at the supraclavicular level with a medium- to high-frequency linear transducer (5-10MHz). The transducer face should be less than 4cm wide to facilitate coupling in the uneven supraclavicular fossa. Obtain a color-flow image of the proximal subclavian vein. Next trace the internal jugular vein upward in transverse section from its confluence with the subclavian vein while applying intermittent compression; follow the vein as far cephalad as possible. If findings are normal (i.e., if the vein is completely compressible), the B-mode image is satisfactory. Now continue the examination below the clavicle. The veins are deeply situated when scanned through the transpectoral window, and therefore a variable-frequency transducer should be set to a low frequency. Starting just below the clavicle, trace the vessels as far as the anterior axillary fold. Then continue scanning through an axillary approach, making certain to overlap the axillary scan with the transpectoral scan to avoid missing portions of the axillary vein. After leaving the axilla peripherally, extend the arm down over the table edge to improve visualization of the veins. If desired, you may try to image the brachiocephalic vein from a supraclavicular approach using a high-frequency transducer. Usually there is no need to examine the forearm.

Figure 89.2 shows the early recanalization of a subclavian thrombosis **(4)**. The scan corresponds to that in **Figure 89.1c**. **Figure 89.3** shows an old subclavian thrombosis. The occluded portion of the vein **(a)** appears to blend with surrounding tissues due to fibrous organization.

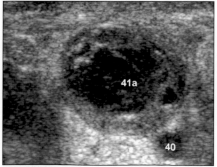

Fig. 89.4a

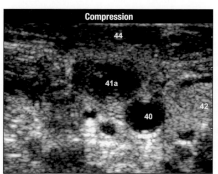

Fig. 89.4b

Figure 89.4a shows a fresh thrombosis of the internal jugular vein **(41a)**. Note how greatly the vein is enlarged in relation to the posteromedial carotid artery **(40)**. Three weeks later **(Fig. 89.4b)** the vein appears less distended.

Critical evaluation

Suspected deep vein thrombosis

The choice of diagnostic procedure depends on availability. CW Doppler is obsolete if one of the two standard procedures-conventional venography and color duplex scanning (CDS) is available. CDS is preferred, as it is noninvasive and generally takes no longer to complete than venography. An experienced examiner can complete a lower extremity examination in approximately 5-10min. This time may be significantly prolonged under difficult examination conditions (about 5-10% of cases). Examination conditions are excellent when all the deep lower extremity veins can be directly visualized in the B-mode image. DVT in the lower leg can also be excluded in these cases. In an unselected population (i.e., under all examination conditions), there is an approximately 10% rate of false-negative color duplex findings in the lower leg. However, in some cases venography may still be inferior to CDS in the lower leg, if an incomplete opacification of the three venous systems in the lower leg occurs due to injection technique. The visualization of muscle groups on venograms is haphazard, and therefore ultrasound is superior for diagnosing the isolated thrombosis of a muscle vein.

Besides the lower leg, the pelvis is another difficult region for ultrasound evaluation. Venography is superior for pelvic vein imaging in healthy subjects, although it can be difficult to interpret the "pseudothrombus artifact" caused by nonopacified blood from the deep femoral vein (↗), great saphenous vein, or internal iliac vein **(Fig. 90.1)**. CDS can provide a valuable adjunct to venography in these cases. If there is extensive thrombosis in the thigh and lower leg, contrast opacification at the pelvic level is usually too weak to confirm or exclude involvement of the pelvic veins. Again, CDS can provide a valuable adjunct. If ultrasound is also equivocal or if the vascular surgeon desires a comprehensive map, CT scanning of the pelvis can define the proximal extent of the thrombosis (⇐ in **Fig. 90.2**). It can be extremely difficult to evaluate for recurrent thrombosis with ultrasound in cases of postthrombotic syndrome. Postthrombotic changes in venous trunks, complex collateral pathways, and the difficulty of distinguishing recent from old changes make venography the standard procedure for this type of investigation.

Suspected valvular incompetence

The extent of saphenous varicosity can be ascertained with a small CW probe. In contrast to CW-Doppler, CDS is better for evaluating secondary or postthrombotic insufficiency of the deep lower extremity veins and for demonstrating incompetent perforators. Venography is still the modality of first choice for the evaluation of perforator insufficiency, however.

Suspected thrombosis of upper extremity veins

CDS is the procedure of choice for determining the cause of unexplained arm swelling. CW Doppler is obsolete if either CDS or venography is available. Venography is superior for mapping collateral channels. But in patients with acute arm swelling and the venographic features of old subclavian thrombosis **(Fig. 90.3a)**, CDS can identify (partial) thrombosis of the collateral circulation **(23)** as the cause of the acute swelling **(Fig. 90.3b)**. B-mode imaging is adequate for the detection or exclusion of jugular vein thrombosis.

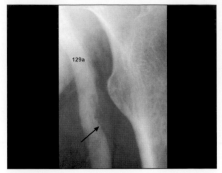

Fig. 90.1

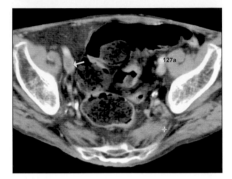

Fig. 90.2

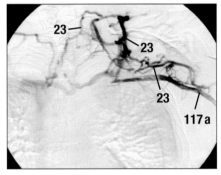

Fig. 90.3a

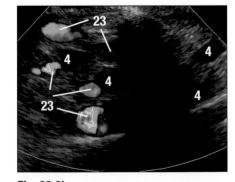

Fig. 90.3b

Quiz – **Take the following quiz to test your knowledge:**

1. What key questions should be answered in the diagnosis of venous thrombosis?
2. What images should be obtained for the minimum documentation of DVT?
3. How is the age of DVT determined with ultrasound?
4. What key questions should be answered in the diagnosis of varicose veins?
5. What is the site of predilection for upper extremity venous thrombosis?

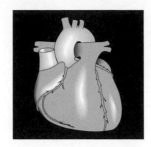

Otto N. Krogmann
Marco Pieper

Introduction

Echocardiography has become the most important tool of the cardiologist for diagnosing significant structural or functional abnormalities of the heart. Anatomic details are accurately portrayed, cardiac structures can be measured and their movements traced throughout the cardiac cycle. Echocardiography thus adds a significant challenge for the investigator compared to ordinary two-dimensional ultrasound imaging of other organs, since the motion of the heart and cardiac segments along the temporal axis yields important functional information. A synchronous electrocardiogram (ECG) is recorded for timing. Of course, this application of ultrasound requires special instrument settings that include a very high temporal resolution (sometimes at the cost of spatial resolution) and a low image persistence.

Besides two-dimensional echocardiography, various methods are available for evaluating the heart and its function:
- One-dimensional M-mode echocardiography for determining sizes (diameters) and evaluating the motion of specific cardiac structures (with high temporal resolution).
- CW Doppler, pulsed Doppler ultrasound or a high pulse repetition frequency (HPRF) for measuring both the velocity and direction of blood flow in the heart and surrounding vessels.
- Color duplex scanning (CDS) for simultaneous two-dimensional color-flow imaging of blood flow velocity and direction.
- Additional studies such as transesophageal echocardiography, contrast echocardiography, and three-dimensional echocardiography are available for special anatomic and functional investigations of the heart.

This chapter cannot replace a complete textbook on echocardiography. Its purpose, rather, is to introduce the reader to the most important imaging planes in echocardiography and demonstrate the value of echocardiography based on several classic pathologic conditions.

Transducer positions

Because the heart is surrounded by ribs and aerated lung tissue, which block the transmission of ultrasound waves, it is best scanned at full expiration from a few selected sites **(Fig. 92.1)**. To make the acoustic windows as large as possible, the patient is placed in a left lateral decubitus position with the upper body slightly elevated. In this position the heart abuts against the anterolateral chest wall and is less obscured by aerated lung, especially at full expiration. Because of the relatively small acoustic window, it is best to use a small sector transducer that produces a pie-shaped scan through the heart. The standard acoustic windows for transthoracic echocardiography are as follows: parasternal in the 2nd-4th intercostal space **(Fig. 92.2 a)**, apical in the 5th or 6th intercostal space **(Fig. 92.2 b)**, suprasternal in the suprasternal notch, and subcostal below the xiphoid process.

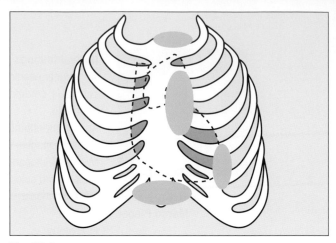

Fig. 92.1

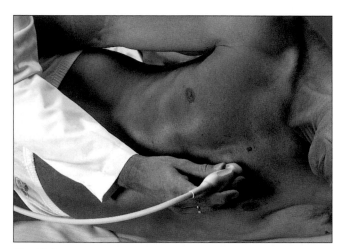

Fig. 92.2 a

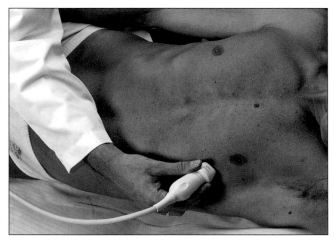

Fig. 92.2 b

Planes of section

By rotating and angling the transducer, the examiner can utilize all the acoustic windows to scan the heart on multiple planes. Three mutually perpendicular planes of section have been defined according to the guidelines of the American Society of Echocardiography: the long-axis view, the short-axis view, and the four-chamber view. The transducer position for these views is based on the axes of the heart, rather than on body axes.

The long axis plane is parallel to the major axis of the heart, defined by a line from the aortic valve to the cardiac apex **(Fig. 92.3a)**. The transducer may be placed in a parasternal, suprasternal, or apical position to obtain a long-axis view. The short axis is perpendicular to the long axis and thus represents a cross-sectional view **(Fig. 92.3b)**. The transducer may be placed in a parasternal or subcostal position. Scanning from the apical or subcostal position provides a four-chamber view that displays all four cardiac chambers in one section **(Fig. 92.3c)**.

The transducer can be angled in both directions to generate additional fan-shaped images through the heart. These special views are particularly useful for the anatomic evaluation of cardiac anomalies. For an accurate analysis of cardiac anatomy and function, the heart should always be scanned in multiple projections and from

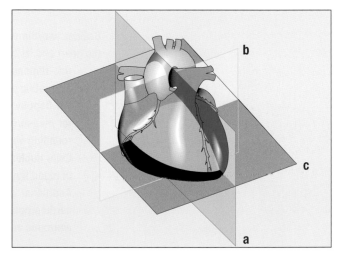

Fig. 92.3

several transducer positions. In this way pathologic structures can be viewed from several angles, they can be fully evaluated, and they can be confidently distinguished from artifacts.

The images that follow are based mainly on three standard planes of section: the parasternal long-axis and short-axis views and the apical four-chamber view.

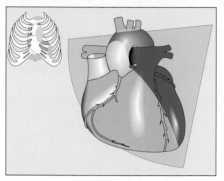

Fig. 93.1a

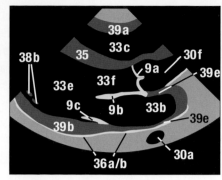

Fig. 93.1b

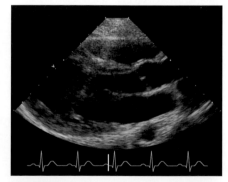

Fig. 93.1c

Parasternal long-axis view

To obtain the parasternal long-axis view, the transducer is positioned in the 3rd or 4th intercostal space anterior to the heart **(Figs. 93.1a, 92.2a)**. The scan plane lies approximately along a line passing from the right shoulder to the left iliac crest. The following structures are visualized from anterior to posterior **(Fig. 93.1b, c)**: the anterior wall of the right ventricle **(39a)**, the right ventricle (outflow tract) **(33c)**, the interventricular septum **(35)**, the left ventricle **(33e)**, and the posterior wall of the left ventricle **(39b)**. Cranial to the left ventricle are the aortic valve **(9a)**, the ascending aorta **(30f)**, the mitral valve **(9b, c)**, the left atrium **(33b)** and, posteriorly, the descending aorta **(30a)**. The correct standard projection is obtained only when all of these structures are simultaneously displayed and the interventricular septum is approximately horizontal. By convention, structures closer to the transducer (right ventricle) are displayed at the top of the image, and cranial structures (aorta) are displayed at the right. Thus, the image is displayed as though the observer were viewing the heart from the left side.

Cardiac cycle

A series of echocardiographic pictures in the parasternal long-axis view can be correlated with the ECG trace to demonstrate the movements of heart structures during specific phases of the cardiac cycle **(Fig. 93.2a-f)**.

At the start of diastole (end of the T wave), the mitral valve opens widely, and blood flows swiftly from the left atrium into the left ventricle, which expands. The aortic valve is closed **(Fig. 93.2a)**. At mid-diastole (between the T and P waves), the pressure is equalized between the atrium and ventricle. There is little or no atrioventricular blood flow, and the mitral valve is in an intermediate position **(Fig. 93.2b)**. At the end of diastole, atrial contraction (P wave) again causes rapid blood flow into the ventricle, and the mitral valve is widely open **(Fig. 93.2c)**. At the start of systole (peak of the R wave), contraction of the ventricle causes the mitral valve to close. The aortic valve remains closed during isovolumetric contraction until the pressure in the left ventricle reaches the aortic level **(Fig. 93.2d)**. As the aortic valve opens, the ejection phase begins and the left ventricle becomes smaller **(Fig. 93.2e)**. At the end of the ejection phase, the aortic valve closes and the left ventricle reaches its smallest volume during the cardiac cycle. The mitral valve remains closed until the end of isovolumetric relaxation **(Fig. 93.2f)**.

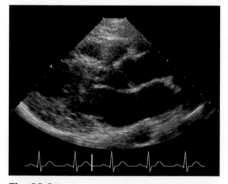

Fig. 93.2a

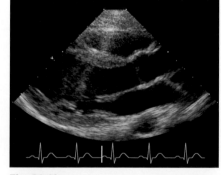

Fig. 93.2b

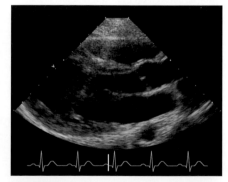

Fig. 93.2c

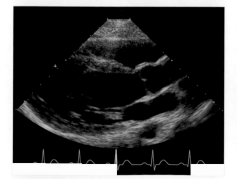

Fig. 93.2d

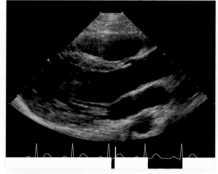

Fig. 93.2e

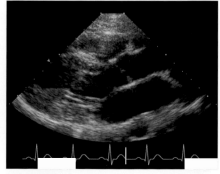

Fig. 93.2f

Parasternal short-axis view

To obtain the parasternal short-axis view, the transducer is again positioned in the 3rd or 4th intercostal space anterior to the heart **(Fig. 94.1)**. The scan plane is perpendicular to the long axis and is displayed as if viewed from below. The transducer can be tilted **(Fig. 94.1b)** to demonstrate various anatomic planes. The lines in the long-axis view in **Figure 94.1c** mark the location of the short-axis planes, which are described below.

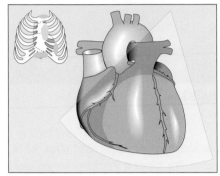

Fig. 94.1a

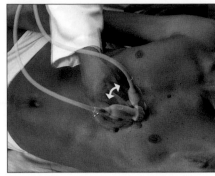

Fig. 94.1b

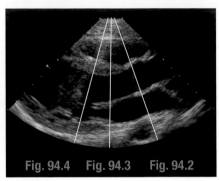

Fig. 94.1c

The vascular plane **(Fig. 94.2)** displays the aortic valve **(9a)** at the center of the image, where its three cusps form a stellate pattern. The curved area anterior to the valve is the right ventricular outflow tract (RVOT) **(33d)**, which connects the inflow tract and tricuspid valve **(9d, left side of image)** with the pulmonary valve **(9e)** and main pulmonary trunk **(155, right side of image)**. Below the aorta is the left atrium **(33b)**.

The mitral valve plane **(Fig. 94.3)** displays the anterior **(9b)** and posterior **(9c)** mitral valve leaflets and the left ventricular outflow tract (LVOT) **(33f)**. The mitral valve leaflets exhibit a distinctive fish-mouth motion during the cardiac cycle.

In the papillary muscle plane **(Fig. 94.4)**, the right ventricle **(33c)** forms a shell-like space at upper left that is anterior to the almost circular left ventricle (LV, **33e**) at the lower right. The two papillary muscles **(38a, b)** appear as posterior structures on the right and left sides.

The concentric contraction of the LV can be clearly observed in the papillary muscle plane during the cardiac cycle. The diastolic image **(Fig. 94.4b)** shows the round LV with the interventricular septum **(35)** and posterior wall **(39b)**.

During systole **(Fig. 94.4a)** the LV cavity becomes smaller, accompanied by a thickening of the septum and posterior wall.

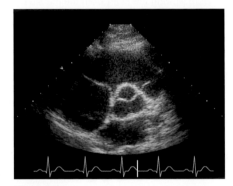

Fig. 94.2 a

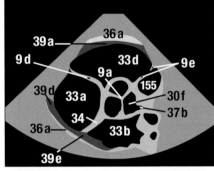

Fig. 94.2 b

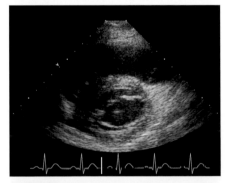

Fig. 94.3 a

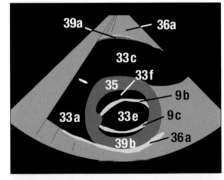

Fig. 94.3 b

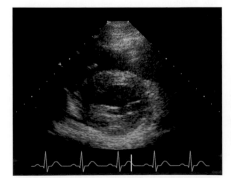

Fig. 94.4 a

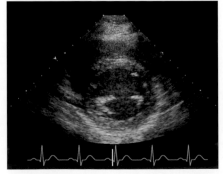

Fig. 94.4 b

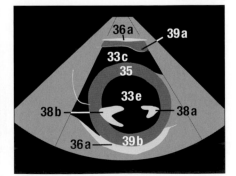

Fig. 94.4 c

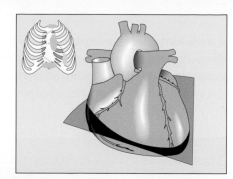

Fig. 95.1

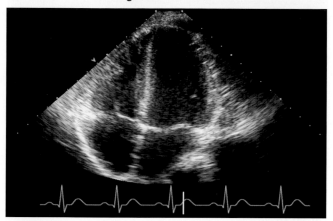

Fig. 95.2 a

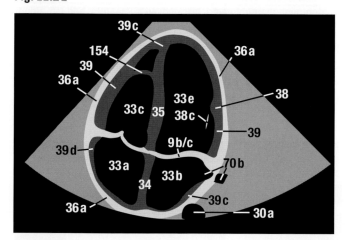

Fig. 95.2 b

Apical four-chamber view

Even in obese patients with a poor acoustic window, a four-chamber view can be obtained from the apical transducer position by scanning through the fifth or sixth intercostal space in left lateral decubitus position (see **Fig. 92.2b**). The beam is aimed toward the right shoulder, transecting the heart from apex to base **(Fig. 95.1)**. Breath-holding at full expiration can enlarge the acoustic window by clearing it of aerated lung. The four-chamber plane is perpendicular to both the long-axis and short-axis planes. The examiner views the heart from below, and thus the positions of the left and right sides of the heart are reversed.

The image is displayed with the cardiac apex **(39c)** at the top (closer to the transducer). The right atrium **(33a)** and right ventricle **(33c)** are to the left **(Fig. 95.2)**. Although effort and patience are needed to obtain this standard view, it displays both atria and ventricles in addition to the atrial septum **(34)**, ventricular septum **(35)**, and both atrioventricular valves **(9)**. The transducer must be accurately positioned over the apex and then rotated and tilted to obtain a precise section that displays all four chambers of the heart. This view is excellent for evaluating the ventricular and atrial septa, the atrioventricular connections, and the function of the chambers.

Five-chamber view

This view is obtained by tilting the transducer anteriorly and rotating clockwise from the apical four-chamber plane to display the left ventricular outflow tract and aortic valve **(Fig. 95.3)**. It is not always easy to define all the structures in the right half of the heart and keep them in view. The scan plane parallels blood flow into the aorta, creating an optimum situation for Doppler imaging of the left ventricular outflow tract **(33f)**, aortic valve **(9a)**, and ascending aorta **(30f)**.

Transoesopageal echocardiography

A poor acoustic window due to obesity or emphysema may not allow adequate visualization of all cardiac structures in transthoracic echocardiography. Transesophageal echocardiography is a good option in such cases, providing an excellent view of the atria, ventricles, and AV valves. It is particularly helpful in the operating room and in the ICU during the early postoperative period after cardiac procedures. A special endoscope with a biplane or multiplane probe is introduced into the hypopharynx and advanced into the esophagus until the heart is seen from behind. The perfect view of the left atrium adjacent to the probe allows for visualization of thrombi in the left atrium or left atrial appendage, the mitral valve, and any defects in the interatrial septum.

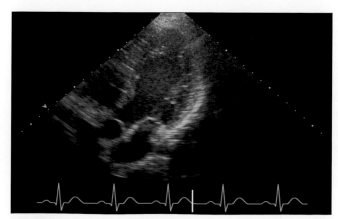

Fig. 95.3 a

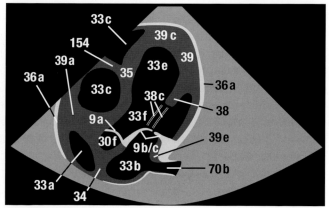

Fig. 95.3 b

M-mode echocardiography

Despite tremendous advances in two-dimensional imaging technology, M-mode (motion) echocardiography is still a fast, simple method for obtaining a global impression of cardiac dimensions and function. Unlike two-dimensional imaging, ultrasound signals are transmitted and received along a single beam to record the movement of cardiac structures. The ultrasound beam is placed in the desired position using the simultaneously displayed two-dimensional image. Changes in wall thickness and chamber sizes as well as valve motion patterns can be displayed and measured with very high temporal resolution. Two projections are illustrated below.

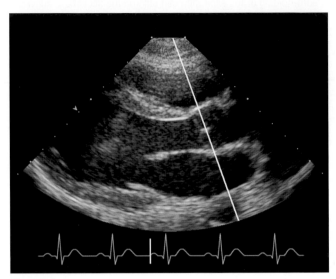

Fig. 96.1a

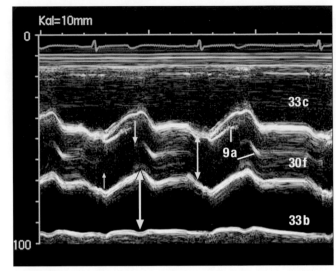

Fig. 96.1b

The first projection is in the long-axis plane. The M-mode beam is directed through the right ventricular outflow tract, aorta, and left atrium at the level of the aortic valve **(Fig. 96.1a)**. The motion pattern of the aortic valve **(9a)** appears at the center of the M-mode display **(Fig. 96.1b)**. The traces below it depict the changing size of the left atrium **(33b)**. The point at which the aortic valve opens (⇑) just past the QRS complex is clearly displayed. Following an ejection phase lasting approximately 0.2 seconds, the aortic valve closes (⇓) and forms a central valve echo. The left atrium below it shows classic size variations during the cardiac cycle, as it becomes larger during ventricular systole and smaller in diastole after closure of the aortic valve. The size of the aorta **(30f, ↕)** is measured at end diastole. The left atrium **(33b, ↕)** is measured at end systole at the point of its maximal expansion.

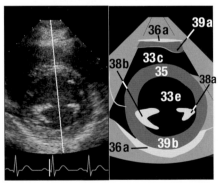

Fig. 96.2a

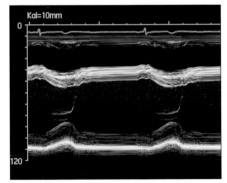

Fig. 96.2b

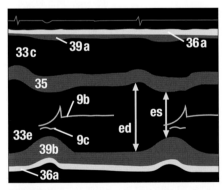

Fig. 96.2c

The second M-mode projection is in a short-axis plane through the left ventricle **(33e)** at the level of the mitral valve chordae **(Fig. 96.2a,b)**. The beam passes transversely through the LV between the two papillary muscles **(38)**, displaying the anterior wall of the right ventricle **(39a)** at the top **(Fig. 96.2c,d)**, then the right ventricle **(33c)**, ventricular septum **(35)**, left ventricular cavity **(33e)**, and the posterior wall of the left ventricle **(39b)**. This view clearly demonstrates that during systole the septum and the left ventricular posterior wall become thicker and the LV cavity smaller. The inner diameter of the LV is measured at end diastole at the start of the QRS complex (↕ **ed**) and at end systole at peak downward displacement of the septum (↕ **es**). The difference between these diameters divided by the end-diastolic diameter, expressed as a percentage, is called fractional shortening (FS) and is an important clinical parameter of LV function **(Table 96.3)**.

Fractional Shortening

$$FS = \frac{(LV_{ed} - LV_{es})}{LV_{ed}} \times 100\%$$

LV_{ed}, LV_{es}: transverse inner diameter of the LV at end diastole and end systole. The normal range of fractional shortening is 28-35%.

Table 96.3

Doppler and color duplex echocardiography

Doppler and color duplex functions make it possible to visualize and quantify blood flow in the heart. They are particularly useful for evaluating the cardiac valves for signs of insufficiency or stenosis. Additionally, the cardiac output can be estimated by measuring flow in the major vessels, and flow abnormalities like those associated with congenital heart defects can be demonstrated (see p.101). Correct adjustment of the standard two-dimensional image is essential for the effective use of Doppler and color duplex functions.

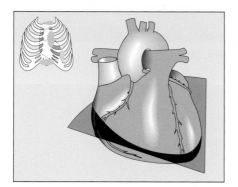

Fig. 97.1a

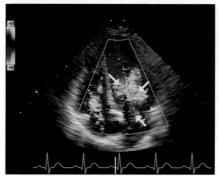

Fig. 97.1b

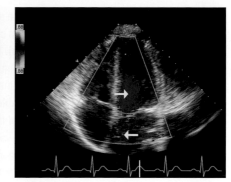

Fig. 97.1c

Atrioventricular valves

The apical acoustic window, especially the four-chamber view **(Fig. 97.1a)**, is best for visualizing blood flow through the AV valves. Normal flow has the following appearance in the color-flow image: after closure of the semilunar valves, the AV valves open in early diastole and blood flows along the pressure gradient between the atria and the relaxed ventricles, covering the full width of the open valve orifices as it enters the ventricles **(Fig. 97.1b)**. The rapid inflow of blood through the mitral valve appears as a cloud of red pixels ( ) with central aliasing (red/blue interface). This causes a redistribution of blood in the left ventricle, as blood in the left ventricular outflow tract flows slowly toward the aortic valve (blue pixels,). Atrial contraction then produces a second phase of ventricular filling. This is followed by closure of the AV valves and the onset of systole. If the valves are intact, no regurgitant flow should occur through the valve leaflets during systole **(Fig. 97.1c)**. There should be only blue-encoded flow in the LVOT directed toward the aortic valve ($\Rightarrow$). The red area ($\Leftarrow$) represents blood entering the left atrium from the pulmonary veins.

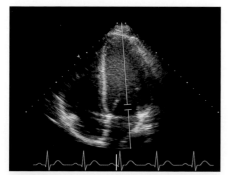

Fig. 97.2

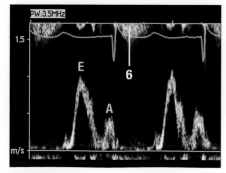

Fig. 97.3

Doppler spectral analysis

A diastolic Doppler spectrum of flow through the AV valve is obtained by positioning the sample volume at the center of the blood stream near the tips of the valve leaflets **(Fig. 97.2)**.

If the sample volume is placed too far toward the ventricular side, the spectrum will show an increase in early diastolic inflow and a decrease in the atrial component.

Correct positioning of the sample volume will yield a normal "M-shaped" Doppler spectrum of the AV valves **(Fig. 97.3)**. The higher initial peak characterizes early diastolic inflow into the relaxed ventricle and is called the E wave (for "early"). The second, smaller peak is produced by atrial contraction and is called the A wave (for "atrial").

The peak velocities of the E and A waves are used to calculate the E/A ratio **(Table 98.5)**. This velocity ratio is age-dependent, being higher in young patients and decreasing with age. It also depends on the heart rate and cardiac output: as the heart rate rises, diastole shortens and therefore atrial contraction contributes more to ventricular filling. This is reflected in the Doppler spectrum by an augmentation of the A wave, causing the E/A ratio to decrease. If the E/A ratio is abnormal with the AV valve being intact, this usually indicates abnormal diastolic ventricular function, i.e., impaired early diastolic relaxation or reduced compliance of the ventricle.

Left ventricular outflow tract and aorta

Blood flow in the LVOT and aortic valve is generally displayed best in the apical five-chamber view (see p.95). The transducer should be positioned so that the beam is approximately parallel to the flow in the LVOT. After an optimum B-mode image has been obtained, color flow can be activated to get an impression of flow characteristics. In normal systole, this will demonstrate laminar flow (✎) away from the transducer in the LVOT and across the aortic valve **(Fig. 98.1)**. The high flow velocity may cause aliasing if the frequency shift exceeds the Nyquist limit (see p.12).

To record a Doppler spectrum, position the sample volume in the aorta directly behind the valve **(Fig. 96.2 a)**. The normal aortic spectrum shows laminar systolic flow into the aorta with a sharp rise and fall in flow velocity **(Fig. 98.2 b)**. In diastole, there should be no regurgitant flow through the valve in either the Doppler spectrum or the color-flow image.

When a spectrum has been recorded from the aortic valve, the cardiac stroke volume can be calculated using the formula shown below **(Table 98.3)**.

VTI (velocity time integral) is the integral of the spectral trace, or the area under the waveform. It can be determined by planimetric analysis. A is the perfused area of the aorta; it can be determined by measuring the diameter of the aortic anulus and using the formula for the area of a circle ($2 \cdot \pi \cdot r^2$). Because the radius is squared, however, even a small error in measuring the radius will lead to a large error in the result.

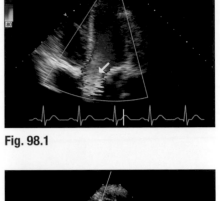

Fig. 98.1

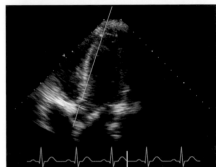

Fig. 98.2 a

Stroke volume of the heart		
SV = A · VTI	SV = stroke volume (ml) VTI = velocity time integral (cm)	A = cross-sectional area of the aorta (cm²)

Table 98.3

Right ventricular outflow tract and pulmonary artery

Blood flow in the RVOT can be evaluated by imaging the pulmonary trunk in a parasternal short-axis view at the level of the aortic root **(Fig. 98.4a)**. The acute beam angle relative to the blood flow is excellent for recording Doppler spectra. As in the aorta, orientation is established by color flow and the pulsed Doppler sample volume is placed at the center of the blood stream, directly behind the open valve **(Fig. 98.4b)**. The spectrum is similar to that in the aorta but with lower peak velocities **(Fig. 98.4c; Table 98.5 [9.1])**.

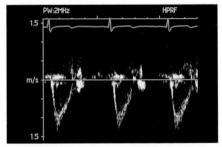

Fig. 98.2 b

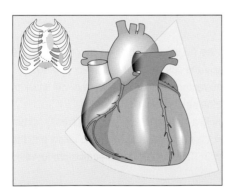

Fig. 98.4 a

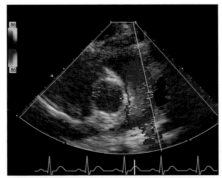

Fig. 98.4 b

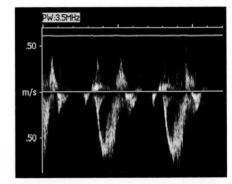

Fig. 98.4 c

Normal peak velocities					
Aorta	1.35 m/sec	1.0-1.7 m/s	**Pulmonary artery**	0.75 m/s	0.6-0.9 m/s
Mitral valve			**Tricuspid valve**		
E wave	0.72 m/sec	± 0.14 m/s	E wave	0.51 m/s	± 0.07 m/s
A wave	0.40 m/sec	± 0.10 m/s	A wave	0.27 m/s	± 0.08 m/s
E/A ratio	1.9	± 0.6	E/A ratio	2.0	± 0.5

Table 98.5

Pathology

Pericardial effusion

Figure 99.1 illustrates the appearance of pericardial effusion in a parasternal long-axis view. Note the echo-free space **(32)** approximately 1-2cm wide surrounding almost the entire heart. Typical features are the acoustic enhancement along the epicardium (↗), the small cavity of the left ventricle, and the apparent left ventricular hypertrophy. In the two-dimensional moving image, the heart appears to float within the effusion.

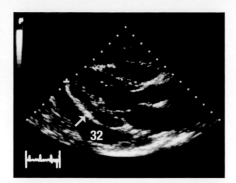

Fig. 99.1

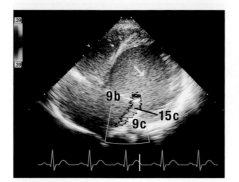

Fig. 99.2

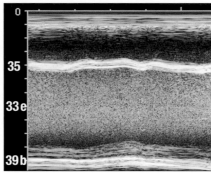

Fig. 99.3

Dilatative cardiomyopathy

Figure 99.2 shows the classic appearance of dilatative cardiomyopathy in the apical four-chamber view. The left ventricle has an enlarged inner diameter and appears more rounded than usual. The low blood flow velocity within the ventricle creates a mottled echo pattern (↘) within the left ventricular cavity. Stretching of the mitral valve ring **(9b, c)** often leads to secondary mitral insufficiency. This is evidenced by high-velocity regurgitant flow **(15c)** through the closed mitral valve into the left atrium, appearing as a predominantly blue jet below the mitral valve.

The M-mode echocardiogram **(Fig. 99.3)** demonstrates the enlarged end-diastolic left ventricular diameter and the lack of motion of the septum **(35)** and posterior wall **(39b)**. The left ventricle in this 10-year-old girl is almost 6cm in diameter and shows only about 15% fractional shortening.

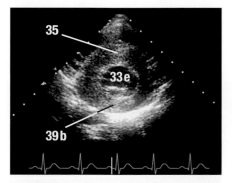

Fig. 99.4

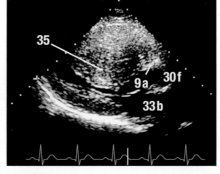

Fig. 99.5

Hypertrophic obstructive cardiomyopathy

The short-axis view in **Figure 99.4** demonstrates severe left ventricular hypertrophy in a patient with hypertrophic cardiomyopathy. The left ventricular cavity **(33e)** is typically small, while the posterior wall of the left ventricle **(39b)** and especially the interventricular septum **(35)** are severely hypertrophic. The changes are even more conspicuous in the long-axis view **(Fig. 99.5)**, which demonstrates the small left ventricular cavity in systole. The hypertrophic septum **(35)** is more than 3cm thick and projects into the left ventricular outflow tract, causing significant obstruction. The aortic valve ring **(9a)** and aorta **(30f)** are of normal size.

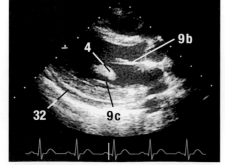

Fig. 99.6

Bacterial endocarditis

The diastolic image on the left **(Fig. 99.6)** is a long-axis view in a patient with bacterial endocarditis. The mitral valve is open. Between the anterior **(9b)** and posterior **(9c)** valve leaflets is a free-floating echogenic structure **(4)** that is adherent to the mitral valve. It represents a large valvular vegetation, which is the hallmark of infective endocarditis. Behind the left ventricle is an effusion **(32)** reflecting pancarditis in this seriously ill patient.

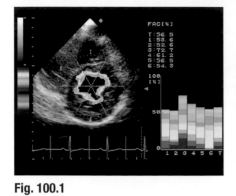

Fig. 100.1

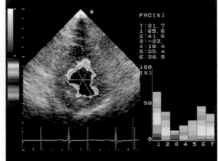

Fig. 100.2

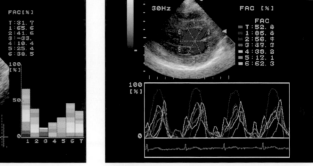

Fig. 100.3

Analysis of wall motion abnormalities

Automatic segmental motion analysis (ASMA) is a relatively new method for evaluating segmental wall motion in the heart. Segmental abnormalities of cardiac contraction are automatically detected and assigned to a specific location in the heart wall. With the aid of a high-resolution digital converter built into the system, the endocardial contours are registered every 40ms during the cardiac cycle and are mapped in a real-time color-coded display. This color representation of segmental wall motion remains on the monitor for a complete cardiac cycle and is refreshed at the start of the next cycle.

Figure 100.1 shows a parasternal short-axis view of the left ventricle in the papillary muscle plane of a healthy subject. End diastole is encoded red, and end systole is encoded blue. The left ventricular cavity is subdivided into six segments so that the contractile motion of each segment can be separately displayed. The end-diastolic and end-systolic segmental areas are used to calculate the fractional area change (**FAC, Table 100.4; Fig. 100.1**), which is compared with the average for all the segments **(T)**. A bar graph indicates the homogeneous contraction of all the wall segments in this normal subject. **Figure 100.2** shows a left ventricle in which global and especially regional wall motion are significantly reduced. Segments 3 and 4, representing the posterior wall of the left ventricle, are the most strongly affected.

The area changes can also be plotted as a time-varying linear graph. Each line color in **Figure 100.3b** represents a different segment in another patient with abnormal wall motion. The increased function in segment 1 (red, FAC=85%) contrasts with the poor function in segment 5 (green, FAC=17%), which shows no contraction in early systole and only a very weak contraction in late systole and early diastole.

Valvular disease

Aortic stenosis

The apical five-chamber view in **Figure 100.5** demonstrates the left ventricle **(33e)**, LVOT, and aortic valve **(9a)**. The valve is thickened, very echogenic, and shows marked limitation of motion. The systolic image shows turbulent flow ( ) in the ascending aorta beyond the aortic valve. There is a mild degree of accompanying mitral insufficiency, evidenced by a small color jet ( ) below the closed mitral valve. The diastolic image **(Fig. 100.6)** additionally shows regurgitant flow **(15c)** in the LVOT as a sign of aortic insufficiency. The patient is an elderly woman with severe, degenerative aortic stenosis. The Doppler gradient is 65 mmHg.

Prosthetic valve

Figure 100.7 shows a four-chamber view in a woman with a Björk-Shiley disk prosthesis for mitral valve replacement. In the diastolic image, the AV valves are open. The metallic prosthetic valve ( ) is strongly echogenic and produces a reverberation artifact **(19)** in the underlying atrium and adjacent acoustic shadows **(18)**. An accelerated flow pattern ( ) from the atrium into the ventricle can be seen to the left and right of the obliquely positioned valvular disk.

Fractional area change (FAC) in echocardiography

$$FAC = \frac{A_{ed} - A_{es}}{A_{ed}} \times 100\,\%$$

FAC = fractional area change
A_{ed} / A_{es} = end-diastolic and end-systolic areas

Table 100.4

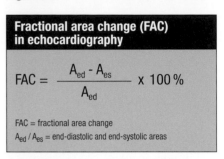

Fig. 100.5

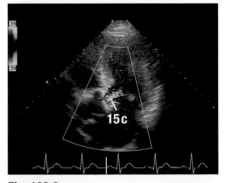

Fig. 100.6

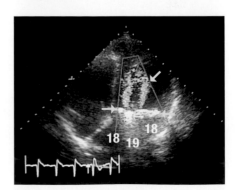

Fig. 100.7

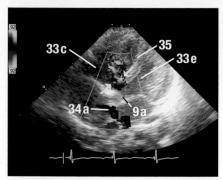

Fig. 101.1

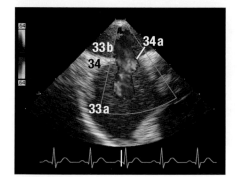

Fig. 101.2

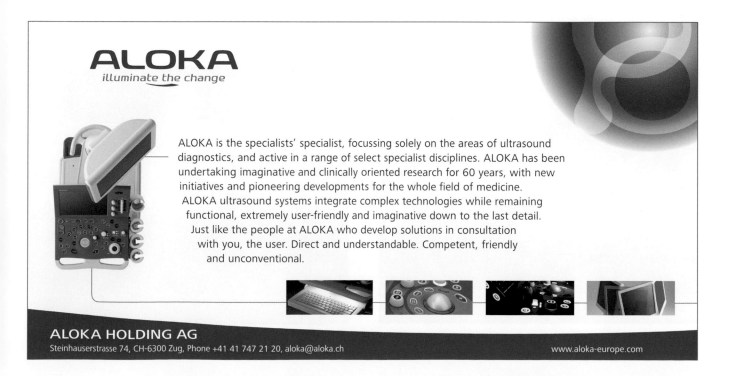

Fig. 101.3

Congenital heart disease

Ventricular septal defect

Figure 101.1 shows a subcostal five-chamber view in a 3-month-old boy with a ventricular septal defect. The defect (↗ ↙) is located in the perimembranous interventricular septum **(35)** directly below the aortic valve **(9a)**. This systolic image shows a conspicuous, red-encoded shunt from the left ventricle to the right ventricle. The atrial septum also contains a small defect **(34a)** through which blood is shunted from the left atrium to the right atrium.

Tetralogy of Fallot

The long-axis view in **Figure 101.2** illustrates the typical features of this anomaly in a 13-year-old girl. The ventricular septum **(35)** between the right ventricle **(33c)** and left ventricle **(33e)** terminates just below the closed aortic valve **(9a)**, leaving an approximately 1-cm defect in the septum. The aortic valve ring is markedly expanded to almost 4cm, and the aorta over-rides the crest of the ventricular septum. The mitral valve is open, and the left atrium **(33b)** is somewhat small. The anterior wall of the right ventricle **(39a)** is as thick as the left ventricular posterior wall **(39b)** as a sign of severe right ventricular hypertrophy.

Atrial septal defect

Figure 101.3 shows an atrial septal defect imaged by transesophageal echocardiography (TEE) using a small probe passed into the esophagus. The advantage of TEE over conventional transthoracic echocardiography lies in the close proximity of the esophagus to the heart. This permits the use of a very high-frequency transducer (5-10MHz), which greatly improves spatial resolution. In TEE the heart is viewed from the posterior aspect, so that the left atrium **(33b)** is displayed at the top of the image and the right atrium **(33a)** at the bottom. The plane transversely intersects the atrial septum **(34)**, which contains a central defect **(34a)**. Blood shunting from the left atrium to the right atrium is encoded blue as it is directed away from the probe. This atrial septal defect is approximately 1cm in diameter.

Tissue doppler

Tissue doppler is a new technique capable of displaying heart wall motion by coding tissue moving away from the probe blue and tissue moving towards the probe red. This is accomplished by different filter settings. Wall motion abnormalities can thus be better detected. This is very useful in coronary artery disease where stress conditions like exercise or dobutamine infusion lead to diminished coronary flow in the affected artery and consequently to regional myocardial dysfunction. The regional wall motion can be compared at rest and during stress, simultaneously displaying the heart cycle during different stages of stress (i.e. different rates of dobutamine infusion).

Tissue doppler can also be used for analyzing longitudinal myocardial function. This is a sensitive marker for early myocardial dysfunction. Longitudinal shortening can best be studied from an apical four chamber view placing the sample volume in the right and left ventricular free wall and the septum. **Fig.102.1a** shows a systolic frame where the septal shortening in systole is coded in red as movement towards the transducer. The diastolic septal lengthening is coded blue in **Fig.102.1b**.

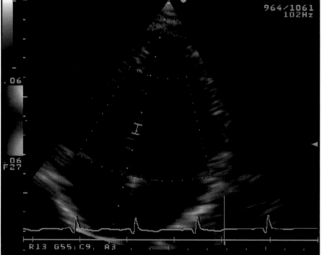

Fig. 102.1a

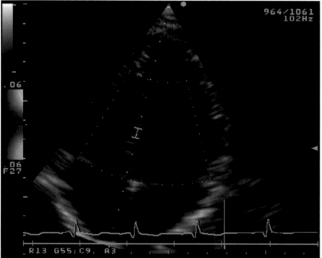

Fig. 102.1b

Myocardial tissue movement can be displayed as a time-velocity graph **(Fig. 102.2 a)** with the normal systolic movement towards the transducer (S-wave) and the diastolic movement from the transducer with an early (E-wave) and a late (atrial, A-wave) peak. In **(Fig. 102.2 b)** the graph shows much less systolic as well as diastolic motion due to a dilative cardiomyopathy in a 38-year-old woman. Note that the E-wave and A-wave have equal amplitudes due to compromised diastolic function (probably delayed relaxation).

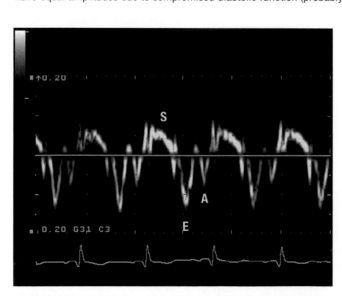

Fig. 102.2 a

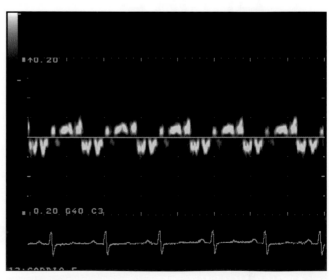

Fig. 102.2 b

Critical evaluation

The enthusiasm for echocardiography is based on the noninvasiveness of the method, which can be used at any time and repeated as often as desired. Today it can provide virtually all information on the anatomy and function of the heart. It can be used in outpatient departments, emergency settings, and even in the operating room or catheterization lab. This broad range of applications is limited only slightly by the fact that echocardiography cannot be used in all patients, due for example to a poor acoustic window, obesity, or pulmonary emphysema. With newer methods such as tissue harmonic imaging, however, image quality in these difficult patients can be substantially improved. Ultrasound contrast agents can also facilitate wall detection. In the apical two-chamber view of the left ventricle and left atrium in **Figure 103.1a**, the lateral endocardium and myocardium are not well defined and the apical region is obscured by artifact. When 0.2 mL of an ultrasound contrast agent is administered and contrast is improved by harmonic imaging, the left ventricular cavity appears white and is easily distinguished from the dark myocardium **(Fig. 103.1b)**. (The two voids represent portions of the suspensory apparatus of the mitral valve.)

Not all cardiac structures (e.g., the coronary arteries and peripheral pulmonary arteries) can be adequately visualized by echocardiography. These vessels require other modalities such as angiography, computed tomography, or magnetic resonance imaging. On the other hand, echocardiography can supply helpful functional information in complex investigations, even though it is often necessary to use additional, somewhat more invasive techniques such as contrast echocardiography, stress echocardiography (exercise or dobutamine), or transesophageal echocardiography.

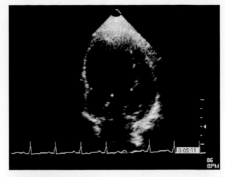

Fig. 103.1a

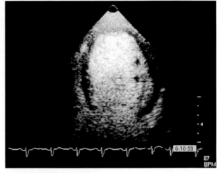

Fig. 103.1b

Recent advances in echocardiographic technology

- The three-dimensional processing of echocardiographic images formerly an off-line, time-consuming, postprocessing task is now available as a real-time tool for the assessment of cardiac structures.
- Coronary artery flow can be visualized by power Doppler echocardiography, and not only in the proximal left and right coronary arteries.
- Color-coded wall motion studies facilitates quick assessment of abnormal regional function.
- Strain and strain-rate imaging, in which myocardial deformation (systolic myocardial shortening and diastolic myocardial lengthening) is imaged independently of global heart movements, yields reliable information on global and regional myocardial function.
- It is reasonable to expect further improvements in the potential applications of echocardiography, giving us a powerful tool for the noninvasive assessment of cardiac morphology and function.

Quiz – Take the following quiz to test your knowledge:

Question 1, see **Abb. 103.2**
    a. What section is displayed?
    b. Do the heart valves, cardiac chambers, and myocardium appear normal?
    c. How would you describe the change in terms of echomorphology?
    d. What is your diagnosis?

Question 2, see **Abb. 103.3**
    a. What section is displayed?
    b. Do the imaged heart structures and blood flow appear normal?
    c. Note the phase of the cardiac cycle in the ECG trace!
    d. What is your diagnosis?

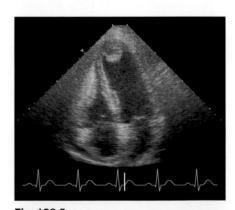

Fig. 103.2

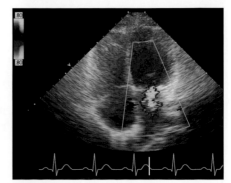

Fig. 103.3

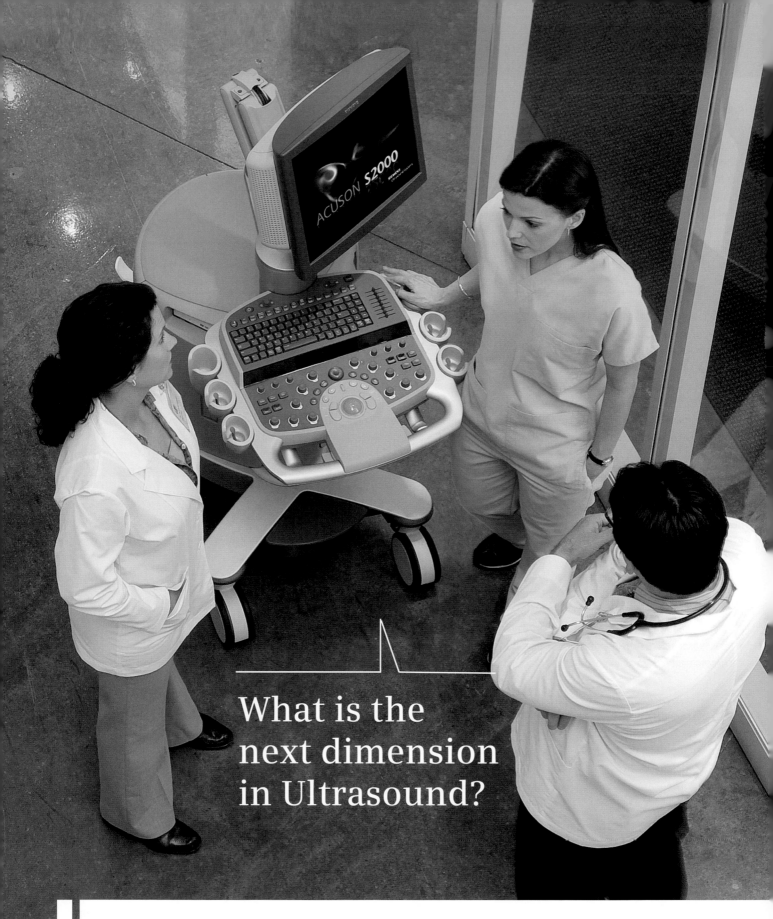

What is the
next dimension
in Ultrasound?

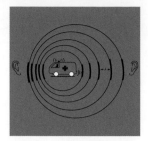

Matthias Hofer

Technical innovations

Introduction

This chapter presents special, but commonly available techniques as well as more recent innovations in the field of diagnostic ultrasound, which have contributed to its diagnostic accuracy and have opened up a broad variety of potential clinical applications. Most of the techniques are named with their general and their product name, given by the first manufacturer, who introduced its use in ultrasound applications. These techniques elucidate the growing relevance of ultrasound as an important diagnostic tool in our daily patient care at present.

Technical innovations

Several technical developments in recent years have brought significant advances in ultrasound image quality and potential new applications for vascular imaging.

Tissue Harmonic Imaging (THI)

This technique does not generate images from the echoes that return to the transducer within the original transmitted frequency band, but utilizes their harmonics – i.e., overtones that are a whole multiple of the fundamental frequency (e.g., 7.0-MHz for a 3.5-MHz source frequency). These harmonics arise only after the beam has reached a certain depth in the tissue **(Fig. 106.1)**, making them immune to the principal causes of image noise and scattering effects that occur at more superficial levels [1.1]. The amplitude of the harmonic signals is significantly lower than the fundamental frequency band, and therefore the fundamental and harmonic imaging bands must be well separated [1.2] **(Fig. 106.2a)**. The 2nd harmonic filtering method separates the frequency bands by using narrow band pulses with lower spatial resolution to avoid an overlap of fundamental and 2nd harmonic frequencies. The phase/pulse-inversion method allows for wideband pulses with better spatial resolution. Although fundamental and harmonic signals overlap, they can be separated by combining the echos of two or more odential transmit pulses that differ only by a phase angle (inversion 180°).

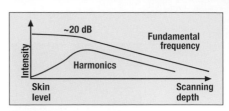

Fig. 106.1

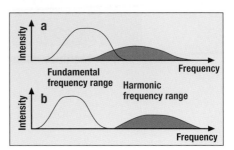

Fig. 106.2

When this condition is satisfied, the harmonic image has a much better signal-to-noise ratio and provides a significant increase in contrast and resolution **(Fig. 106.3b)** compared with conventional imaging **(Fig. 106.3a)**. In the example shown, harmonic imaging makes it easier to classify the upper outline of a cyst as "well-defined" (⬎), and acoustic shadows (⬆) from intrarenal calcifications **(Fig. 106.3b)** would not have been seen with conventional imaging **(Fig. 106.3a)**. In another example, an intravascular thrombus (⬇) at the carotid bifurcation **(Fig. 106.4b)** is clearly demonstrated by harmonic imaging but might have been overlooked with conventional imaging **(Fig. 106.4a)**. This technique is also called second harmonic imaging and can be combined with ultrasound contrast agents (see p. 107). **Figure 107.4b** shows the effect of combining harmonic imaging with contrast administration. The contrast-enhanced study reveals subtle, diffuse metastatic liver disease, which had not been visible on conventional ultrasound scans **(Fig. 107.4a)**.

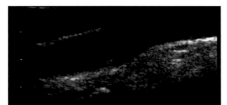

Fig. 106.4a

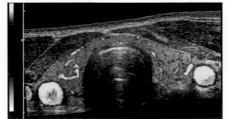

Fig. 106.4b

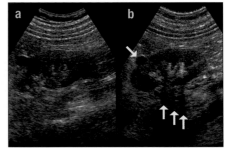

Fig. 106.3

Power Doppler (angio mode)

This technique is based on the energy amplitude of the reflected frequency spectrum and disregards the frequency shift. Thus, while power Doppler provides no information on flow direction or velocity, it is a very sensitive technique for imaging slow flows, small vessel lumina, and parenchymal perfusion **(Fig. 106.5)**. It is less angle-dependent than conventional Doppler, but it is less accurate then conventional color Doppler with PW frequency analysis in the quantification of stenosis.

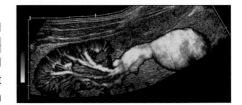

Fig. 106.5

SieScape® Imaging

New high-performance image processors have made it possible to generate real-time ultrasound images up to 60cm long [1.3] by sweeping the transducer slowly and steadily over the body region of interest **(Fig. 106.6)**. With some practice, the examiner can obtain distortion-free panoramic images even along curved skin surfaces **(Fig. 106.7)**. Distance measurements on SieScape® images can be performed to an accuracy of 1-3% [1.4]. **Figure 106.8** shows a septated hydrocele in its largest dimension. SieScape® is also useful in this case for comparing the affected side with the normal right testicle.

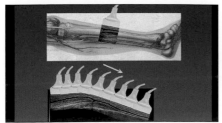

Fig. 106.6

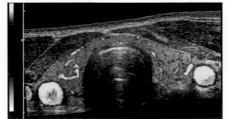

Fig. 106.7

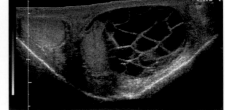

Fig. 106.8

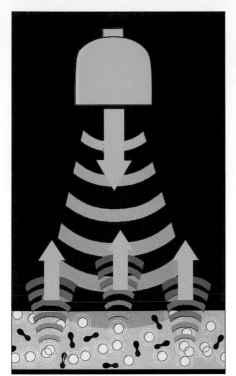

Fig. 107.1

Ultrasound contrast agents

The use of contrast agents for ultrasound signal enhancement is based on the introduction of microbubbles approximately 3-10μm in diameter into the bloodstream. The acoustic impedance mismatch at the surface of the microbubbles greatly amplifies the intensity of the Doppler signals that are returned from the blood **(Fig. 107.1)**. Especially when scanning at greater depths, in obese patients, or when scanning the circle of Willis through a thick temporal bone (see **Fig. 28.3**), this signal enhancement can often permit a diagnosis to be made that would not be possible on unenhanced images. The best results are achieved when echo enhancement is combined with power Doppler and harmonic imaging (see above). Several contrast agents are available:

Levovist® can survive the cardiopulmonary circulation with fractionated i.v. injection and will boost the Doppler signal intensity by 20-25 dB for approximately 10min. It consists of microbubbles (✶) stabilized with a fine palmitic acid coating. The microbubbles average 3μm in diameter, and 95% are smaller than 10μm. Initially, they are bound to galactose microparticles, which dissolve in the bloodstream and release the microspheres **(Fig. 107.2)**. Levovist is usually used with a high mechanical index (MI) above 1.0. The suspension is shaken for 10s, let stand for 2 min, and must be used within the next 8 min.

Another agent, Sonovue consists of an aqueous solution of sulfur hexafluoride microbubbles stabilized by a phospholipid film [1.6] and is used with low MI-values (mechanical index below 0.1). The microbubbles average 2.5 μm in size (90% < 8 μm) and have an osmolality of 290 mosmol/kg **(Fig. 107.3)**. The suspension is convenient to use, as it remains stable for 6 hours. Its echo-enhancing properties are illustrated in **Figure 82.1**.

Note again the benefit of combining tissue harmonic imaging with contrast agents in the detection of subtle metastatic liver disease **(Fig. 107.4)**.

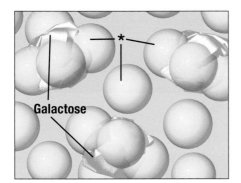

Fig. 107.2

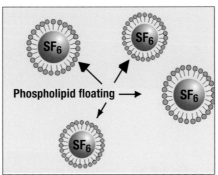

Fig. 107.3

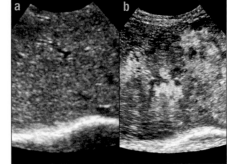

Fig. 107.4

Clarify® vascular enhancement technology

This technology is based on an algorithm that can significantly reduce B-mode image unsharpness caused by partial-volume and beam-width effects. It uses flow information derived from power Doppler to enhance the spatial resolution of vascular margins in the B-mode display.

This technology improves our ability to detect soft- and hard-plaque contours in the carotid arteries, for example **(Fig. 107.5b)**, compared with the normal display in **Figure 107.5a**. In studies of peripheral liver vascularity, Clarify® can significantly improve luminal definition of the hepatic veins and portal venous branches in the hepatic parenchyma **(Fig. 107.6)**.

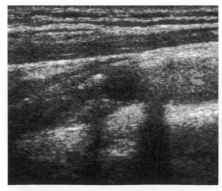

Fig. 107.5a Conventional B-mode image of the carotid artery

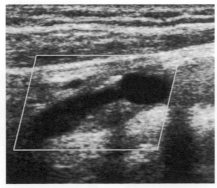

Fig. 107.5b with Clarify® vascular enhancement technology

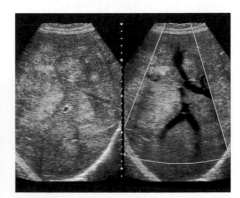

Fig. 107.6 Hepatic vessels

Pulse compression

This procedure, which is derived from radar technology, is primarily used for better visualization of deep structures. Given the potential for thermal and mechanical damage, it is not possible to increase penetration simply by increasing pulse transmission. The transmitted pulses may be lengthened, however, and their frequency modulated according to a certain pattern ("chirp coding"). A single transmitted pulse thus contains more energy while maintaining the same amplitude **(Fig. 108.1a)**. The reflected echoes are then decoded by a chirp receiver and converted into shorter echoes with a correspondingly higher amplitude **(Fig. 108.1b)**.

This increases penetration without the loss of detail that occurs at lower frequencies and that results in poorer resolution. **Figure 108.2c** shows a hypoechoic mass **(29)** behind the thyroid **(42)**, which would have gone undetected without pulse compression **(Fig. 108.2a)**.

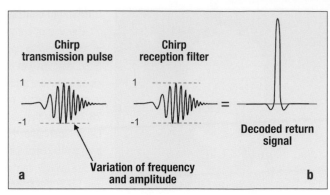

Fig. 108.1

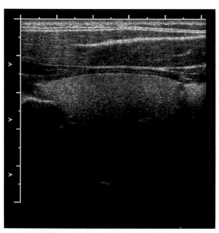

Fig. 108.2a

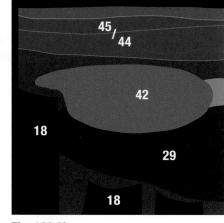

Fig. 108.2b

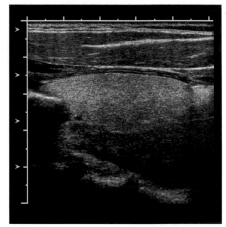

Fig. 108.2c

Precision upsampling

Using conventional digital imaging techniques, high-frequency transducers receive reflected echoes only 2- to 5-times as fast as the maximum frequency components of the echo (wide grid shown in **Fig. 108.3a**). The reflected echoes are thus usually plotted on only a few points, producing an image that is a mere approximation of the actual echo **(Fig. 108.4a)**. Complex regression algorithms can be used for a much more accurate display of the echo in terms of time and amplitude (narrower grid in **Fig. 108.3b**). This allows, for example, one of the radial tendons (⇑) to be visualized much more clearly **(Fig. 108.4b)**.

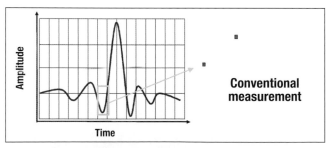

Fig. 108.3a

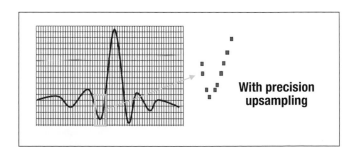

Fig. 108.3b

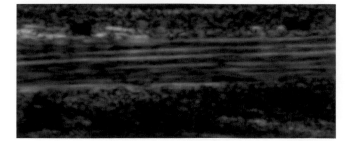

Fig. 108.4a

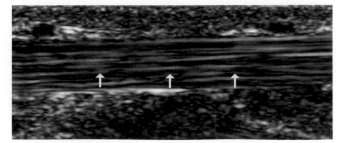

Fig. 108.4b

Diagnostic ultrasound catheter

Another new development are miniature transducers, which are now available in 3-mm-wide catheters that can be rotated 160° in any direction **(Fig. 109.1)**. **Figure 109.2** shows the impressive comparison in size between the AcuNav probe (= accurate navigation, Siemens) and a transesophageal echocardiography (TEE) probe as used in the esophagus. The small expansion of the disposable catheter also enables placement in the heart through the venous system.

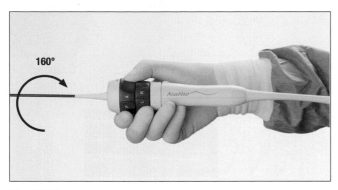

Fig. 109.1

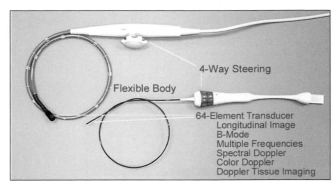

Fig. 109.2

An atrial septal defect (⬇), which was previously difficult to access, can now be much more accurately depicted in B-mode **(Fig. 109.3a)** at much higher frequencies of about 7.5 MHz. The subsequent shunt inflow through the septum is also better visualized on a color flow image **(Fig. 109.3b)** than was generally previously possible. The monitoring of instrumental closure of the ASD (✔ in **Fig. 109.3c**) and assessment of treatment success are also facilitated. Along with superior image quality, the main advantage over TEE is that a sedative or anesthesia is not required, allowing the patient to cooperate during the examination (breath-hold, Valsalva test, etc.) and, on the whole, making the procedure easier for the patient.

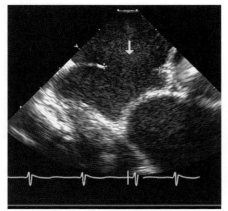

Fig. 109.3a

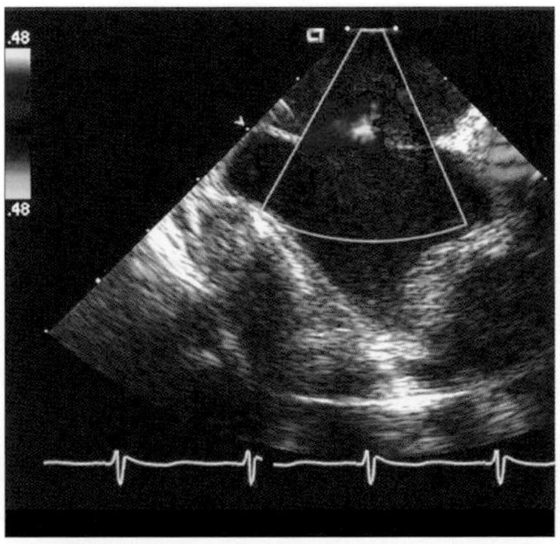

Fig. 109.3b

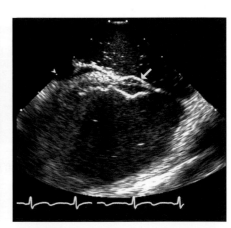

Fig. 109.3c

The catheter may also be advanced through the right heart into the inferior vena cava (IVC), where it may be used to guide direct intrahepatic portocaval shunt (DIPS). From the IVC, adjacent esophageal varices (↘ in **Fig. 109.4**) and retroperitoneal lymph nodes **(50)** are depicted with very high local resolution **(Fig. 109.5)**. The image shows the development of necrosis **(109)**. Note also the precise depiction of the layers of the wall (⟹) of the neighboring duodenum **(80b)**.

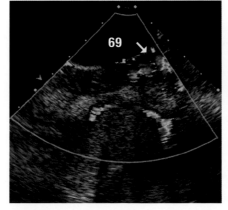

Fig. 109.4

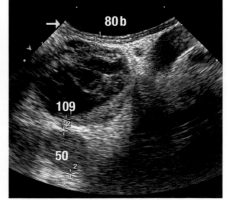

Fig. 109.5

Automated measurements of IMT and vessel wall stiffness

Numerous studies have shown that the intima-media thickness (IMT, see pp. 23/24) correlates with the risk of cardiovascular events (myocardial infarction, stroke). As the walls of arterial vessels undergo increasing fat accumulation and calcification, they become stiffer in response to the fluctuating pressures generated by arterial pulse waves [1.8].

When we compare the compliance of healthy vessels **(Fig. 110.1a)** with that of stiffened vessels **(Fig. 110.1b)**, we find that for equal pulse-wave amplitudes, the stiffer vessels undergo a smaller relative increase in vascular diameter during systole **(Fig. 110.2)**. In the example shown in **Figure 110.1**, the relative increase is 8% in a normal vessel and less than 4% in a stiffened vessel.

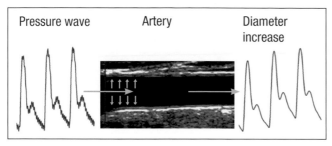

Fig. 110.1a Normal vessel

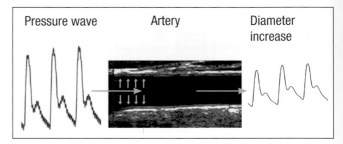

Fig. 110.1b Stiffened vessel wall

Several manufacturers offer automated ultrasound programs that can measure the position of the near and far vessel walls over time with high precision for the determination of vessel wall compliance and pulse wave velocity (PWV).

The most useful programs are those that display quality indicators during the measurement, enabling the examiner to optimize the probe position during the study and define a section passing through the exact center of the vessel lumen **(Fig. 110.3)**.

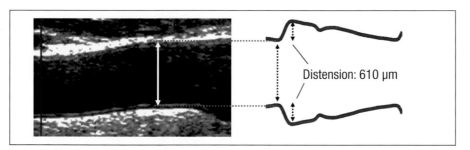

Distension: 610 μm

Fig. 110.2 Increase in vessel diameter in μm during systole

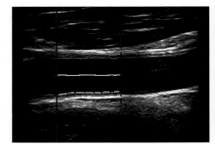

Fig. 110.3 Automatic measurement of compliance (stiffness)

High-Resolution Color Doppler Techniques

The power Doppler technique (see p. 106) has been further developed by various manufacturers with the aim of visualizing the actual vascular lumina with greater precision **(Fig. 111.1)** and over a broader area **(Fig. 111.2)**. Several modern devices employing this technique achieve very high spatial resolution (< 0.3 mm). Various proprietary systems implement these techniques under trade names such as "eFLOW", "Dynamic Flow", and "Clarify Vascular Enhancement Technology" (see p. 107). They are very well suited for visualizing the complex vascularization of an organ **(Fig. 111.3)**. These techniques are made possible by modern pulse generators (beam formers) that optimize pulses by shortening transient and decay times. The resulting pulses are extremely short and permit higher spatial resolution. This is a great advantage in evaluating stenosis and organ perfusion.

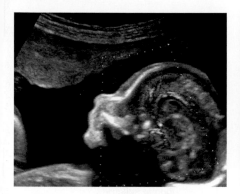

Fig. 111.1 Small vascular lumina

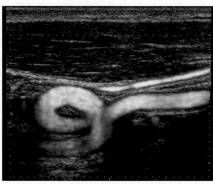

Fig. 111.2 CCA-loop on eFlow

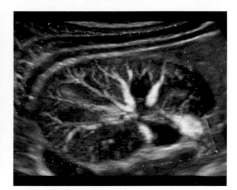

Fig. 111.3 Renal perfusion

Analysis of Vascular Distension (Arterial Stiffness, Echo Tracking, eTracking)

The research on possible causes of cardiovascular disease increasingly focuses on vascular function and vascular mechanics as indicators of the progression or prognosis of these disorders [10.1, 10.2]: Ultrasound measurements of vascular distension can be used to calculate several relevant parameters such as pulse wave velocity (PWV), vascular elasticity (ß index), augmentation index (AI), elastic or "Young's" modulus (EP), and endothelial function (FMD = flow mediated dilation; **Fig. 111.4**). Special software can capture the motion of organ structures by tracking movement of user-defined points along a line of the image (eTracking, **Fig. 111.5**). This is now possible at high temporal resolution (1 KHz) as well as high spatial resolution ($1/16$ of wavelength λ).

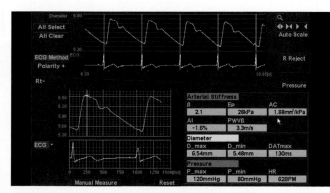

Fig. 111.4 Average of multiple distension cycles (three in this case) over time

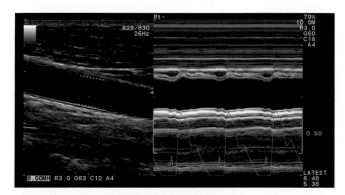

Fig. 111.5 eTracking of CCA distension on ultrasound (l) and M-mode (r)

One extension of this analytical method is based on simultaneous Doppler measurements of blood flow velocity at a single location. This can be used to calculate values such as pulse wave propagation or wave intensity (dP*dU), which describe the link between the heart and the downstream vascular system.

Critical evaluation

We have already mentioned several pitfalls relating to the examiner-dependence of color duplex. Valid results require careful adjustment of all instrument parameters combined with optimum positioning of the ultrasound beam in relation to the vessel of interest. This dependence on the diligence and experience of the examiner is probably the most serious limitation of CDS.

We suggest, therefore, that you review the contents of this introductory chapter before proceeding to Chapter 2, and that you repeat this process for all the chapters that follow. The answers to the self-test quiz can be found on the preceding pages 8 -18 or in the answer keys at the back of the book. Write your answers in the shaded boxes.

Quiz – Take the following quiz to test your knowledge:

1. Define the terms PRF and aliasing.

2. What is the recommended sequence of steps for adjusting the B-mode image, color flow, and pulsed Doppler spectrum? Explain why, for example, you would not adjust the PRF before adjusting the angle of the color box .

3. What are the three main causes of a poor color-flow image in an artery with normal flow?

4. What are the three main causes of a poor color-flow image in veins with normal flow?

5. How do ultrasound contrast agents produce signal enhancement in CDS? What technique can be combined with contrast agents to improve image quality?

Q

Chapter 1/10
Basic physical/New techniques

Question 1 (p.112):

Pulse repetition frequency (PRF) is the rate at which ultrasound pulses are emitted from the transducer per unit time. Aliasing is spurious Doppler shift information, which appears as a mixture of bright colors in the color-flow image or as a cutoff of the spectral waveform. It occurs when the maximum true frequency shift exceeds the Nyquist limit of PRF/2 at high velocities. Ways to compensate for aliasing are listed in **Table 12.4**.

Question 2 (p.112):

Sequence of steps:

B-mode

Step 1:   Angle the probe relative to the vessel axis

Step 2:   Place just one focal zone at the center of the vessel lumen

Step 3:   Set the B-mode gain to a low level

Color flow

Step 4:   Use beam steering to improve the beam-vessel angle (angled away from 90°, see p. 8)

Step 5:   Adjust the PRF to the prevailing flow velocity

Step 6:   Increase the color gain until blooming occurs, then lower the gain until color signals are confined to the vessel lumen (no extravascular color pixels)

Doppler spectrum

Step 7:   Position the sample volume (SV) at the center of the vessel and set the SV size at $^1/_2$ to $^2/_3$ of the luminal diameter

Step 8:   Adjust the baseline level for spectral components above or below the baseline to eliminate waveform cutoff at the top or bottom

Step 9:   Adjust the velocity range (PRF_{PW}). If aliasing still occurs:

Doppler trace too short => $PRF_{PW} \Downarrow$ => to expand the trace vertically
Doppler trace too high => $PRF_{PW} \Uparrow$ => to compress the trace vertically

Step 10: Adjust the PW gain to obtain a good contrast-to-noise ratio: Try to get a dark background without noise pixels, but do not set the gain too low (for automatic envelope curve detection)

Step 11: Remember to enter the insonation angle!

Question 3 (p. 112):

Most common causes of a poor color-flow image in arteries:

☐ Setting the B-mode gain too high
☐ Insonating the vessel at too high an angle
☐ Setting the color gain too low

Question 4 (p. 112):

Most common causes of a poor color-flow image in veins:

☐ Setting the PRF too high
☐ Setting the wall filter too high
☐ Insonating the vessel at too high an angle
☐ Use beam steering!

Question 5 (p. 112):

Contrast agents introduce microbubbles into the blood stream. A very high impedance mismatch develops at the surface of microspheres, increasing the intensity of the echo return by up to 20 dB. Contrast agents are most effective when combined with power Doppler and harmonic imaging.

Chapter 2 Cerebrovascular imaging

Question 1 and 2 (p. 28):
See page 20

Chapter 3 Thyroid

Question 1 (p. 34):
See the tables on pp. 30-31

Question 2 (p. 34):

a.   Diffusely hypoechoic goiter with very heavy, diffuse hypervascularity

b.   Diffusely hypoechoic goiter with moderate hypervascularity

c.   Irregular hypoechoic areas with moderate hypervascularity

d.   Nodular masses of varying echogenicity, with or without a halo, and usually showing peripheral rather than central vascularity

Question 3 (p. 34):
Graves' disease.

Question 4 (p. 34):
Fig. 34.3 see **Table 31.3**
Fig. 34.4 see **Table 31.1**

Chapter 4 Abdomen

Question 1 (p. 48 / Fig. 48.1):

1.   Plane: transverse section through the upper abdomen

2.   Landmarks: aorta **(30b)**, IVC **(76)**, celiac trunk **(71)**, common hepatic artery **(67a)**, splenic artery **(71c)**, liver **(60)**, vertebral body **(21b)**

3.   Display modes: color flow (at left and center of image) and power mode (at upper right)

4.   See the table below

5.   Flow phenomena: flow reversal in the celiac trunk, aliasing

6.   Suspicious findings: dilatation of the celiac trunk, aliasing

7.   Diagnosis: celiac trunk aneurysm due to poststenotic dilatation

Flow direction	Vessels
Toward the transducer	Aorta, celiac trunk, proximal CHA, proximal splenic artery
Away from the transducer	IVC, distal splenic artery, distal CHA

Q

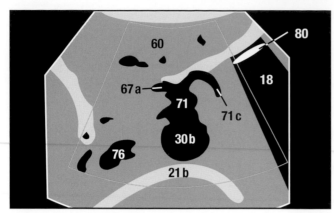

Diagram for answers 1–4

Question 2 (p. 48 / Fig. 48.2):

1. Plane: transverse section just above the aortic bifurcation
2. Landmark: aorta
3. Display mode: color flow
4. Vessels, flow direction: aorta
5. Measurements: diameters of the total lumen and perfused lumen
6. Suspicious finding: eccentric lumen with irregular perfusion
7. Diagnosis: partially thrombosed abdominal aortic aneurysm with risk of rupture

Chapter 5 Nephrology and urology

Question 1 (p. 62):

The RI in the interlobar arteries and poststenotic kidney is > 0.05 lower than on the opposite side.

Question 2 (p. 62):

Velocities higher than 200 cm/s are suspicious for renal artery stenosis.

Question 3 (p. 62):

There is a high index of suspicion for bilateral RAS, as 0.50 is well below the age-normal range of 0.707–0.855 for a 80 years old patient (see **Table 51.2b**).

Question 4 (p. 62):

The proximal flow velocity is normal (113 cm/s). Color flow shows turbulence (arrow) in the midportion of the renal artery with a flow velocity of 210 cm/s, indicating a stenosis of the middle third of the right renal artery.

Question 5 (p. 62):

The image demonstrates the inferior portion of the testis **(97)** and the tail of the epididymis **(97a)**, which shows markedly increased perfusion. Examination of the asymptomatic side in this patient showed scant flow in the epididymis. Diagnosis: left-sided epididymitis.

Question 6 (p. 62):

The scan shows a normal-appearing testis **(97)** and an abnormal-appearing, nonhomogeneous epididymis **(97a)** with cystic components **(110)**. The scant perfusion in the color-flow image does not support the diagnosis of an acute inflammatory process. The differential diagnosis should include chronic inflammation (specific or nonspecific) and an epididymal tumor (rare!). Histologic examination of the surgical specimen revealed a chronic granulomatous, necrotizing arteritis of the epididymis (also rare!).

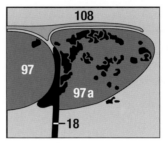
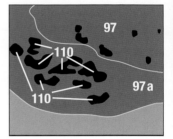

Diagram for answer 5 **Diagram for answer 6**

Chapter 6 Obstetrics and gynecology

Question 1 (p. 74):

Main indications: fetal growth retardation, fetal anomaly, pregnancy-induced hypertension, preeclampsia, diabetes mellitus, etc.

Question 2 (p. 74):

The CPR describes the distribution of blood volume between the fetal brain and the placenta. This parameter is very sensitive for the detection of IUGR. The normal value is >1.

Question 3 (p. 74):

Figure 74.3 shows a nonhomogeneous cystic-solid mass (2 points) with an irregular inner margin (2 points). The solid area is homogeneous (1 point). This gives an ultrasound score of 5, which is in the suspicious range. Color duplex scanning would not be particularly helpful in this case (leukocytosis, second phase of the menstrual cycle). The differential diagnosis should include corpus luteum, but the most likely diagnosis is tuboovarian abscess. Recommenda-tion: antibiotic therapy, follow-up at one week.

Question 4 (p. 74):

The oligohydramnios, IUGR, and abnormal spectrum from the placental vessels are consistent with severe placental insufficiency. Duplex examination should be extended to include the MCA, umbilical vein, ductus venosus, and possibly the aorta to better evaluate the condition of the fetus. We would also recommend a detailed screening evaluation for fetal anomalies (to exclude a fetal heart defect), which may include karyotyping.

Reflux into the umbilical artery warrants immediate referral to a perinatal center. Important: start RSD prophylaxis (pulmonary maturation) right away!

Q

Chapter 7 Peripheral arteries

Question 1 (p. 82):

The scan demonstrates an occlusion of the superficial femoral artery with filiform residual flow. The "stenosis" is the start of a collateral circuit. The intrastenotic increase in PSV by >250% (b) is typical. The poststenotic spectrum (c) shows continuous diastolic forward flow with a small PSV due to the decreased peripheral resistance past the stenosis. Multilevel disease with more proximal stenoses accounts for the decrease in the prestenotic PSV (a).

The different scales used for the spectra provide a clue to the correct solution.

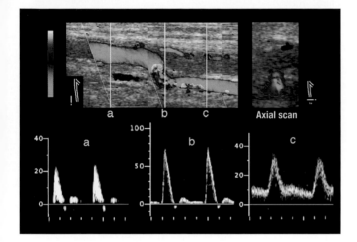

Chapter 8 Peripheral veins

Question 1 (p. 90):

a. Is thrombosis present?
b. What is the extent of the thrombosis?
c. How old is the thrombosis?
d. Is the thrombus adherent to the vessel wall?
e. Does the thrombosis have a detectable cause?

Question 2 (p. 90):

Transverse and longitudinal color-flow images should be obtained to document the cranial end of the thrombus. B-mode images are adequate for comparing the size of the thrombosed vein and accompanying artery in transverse section.

Question 3 (p. 90):

With a fresh lower extremity thrombosis (< 10 days old), the transverse diameter of the thrombosed vein is more than twice the diameter of the accompanying artery.

Question 4 (p. 90):

a. Is venous insufficiency present?
b. What are the proximal and distal limits of the venous insufficiency?
c. Are there anatomic variants at the saphenopopliteal junction?
d. Is the deep venous system patent and competent?

Question 5 (p. 90):

The subclavian vein.

Chapter 9 Echokardiographie

Question 1 (p. 103):

Figure 103.2 shows an apical four-chamber view during systole (ECG: start of T wave, AV valves closed). The atria (**33 a, b**), AV valves (**9 b-d**), and right ventricle (**33 c**) appear normal. The left ventricle (**33 e**) appears dilated, particularly in its apical portion and free wall (arrows). The moving image indicated hypokinesia. The hyperechoic, homogeneous, well-defined rounded structure (**4**) near the apex is a thrombus that formed due to abnormal left ventricular wall motion (e.g., after myocardial infarction). The clot should be imaged in multiple planes. Large, echogenic, mobile thrombi are easier to detect than mural thrombi that show only slightly increased echogenicity. These thrombi are sometimes difficult to distinguish from artifacts.

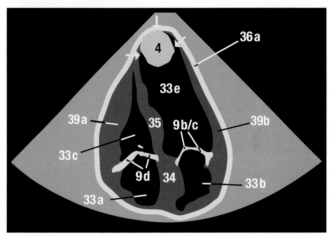

Fig. 103.2b: Diagram for answer 1

Question 2 (p. 103):

Figure 103.3 is an apical four-chamber view. The left and right atria and ventricles exhibit normal morphologic features. The color-flow sector shows rapid, turbulent flow through the closed mitral valve. This flow is predominantly blue and therefore is directed from the left ventricle into the left atrium. The synchronous ECG trace shows that the image was acquired during systole (at the end of the T wave), when there should be no flow through the closed leaflets. This justifies a diagnosis of mitral insufficiency. The etiology of the valvular defect cannot be determined from the echocardiogram alone. The dark blue color in the left ventricle near the septum represents systolic blood flow in the LVOT directed toward the aorta.

Q

Chapter 1+10 / Basic physical and technical principles / Technical innovations

[1.1] **Haberkorn U, Rudat V, Leier G** et al: Der Einfluß von Bauchwandzusammensetzung und Bauchwanddicke auf das Ultraschall B-Bild. Röfo 155 (1991): 327-331

[1.2] **Schoelgens C**: Verbesserung der B-Bild-Diagnostik mit Harmonic Imaging. Ultraschall in Med 5 (1998)

[1.3] **von Behren P, Gustafson D, Haerten R** et al: Neue Entwicklungen in der Ultraschall-Bildgebung mit schneller Multimedia-Technik. Ultrasch in Med 17 (1996): 9

[1.4] **Rosenthal SJ, Lowery CM, Wetzel LH**: Klinische Ultraschallbildtechnik mit SieScape. Electromedica 65 (1997): 15-19

[1.5] **Kempf C.**: The safety of Albumin SRK in terms of virus transmission. Haemo (1997); Haemo Central Laboratory Blood Transfusion Service Swiss Red Cross April 1997

[1.6] **Schneider M, Arditi M, Barrau MB** et al: A new ultrasonographic contrast agent based on sulfur hexafluoride-filledmicrobubbles. Invest Radiol 30 (1995): 451-457

[1.7] **Elsmann BHP, Legemate DA, van der Heyden FWHM** et al: The use of Color-Duplex Scanning in the selection of patients with lower extremity arterial Disease for percutaneous transluminal angioplasty: A prospective study. Cardiovasc Intervent Radiol 19 (1996): 313-316

[1.8] **Laurent S, Cockroft J, Van Bortel L et al.** Expert consensus document on arterial stiffness: methodological issues and clinical applications. Eur Heart J (2006) 27: 2588-2605

Chapter 2 / Cerebrovascular imaging

[2.1] **Hofer M**: Sonographie Grundkurs. Georg Thieme Verlag, Stuttgart, 4. Aufl. (2002): 102

[2.2] **North American Symptomatic Carotid Endarterectomy Trial (NASCET) Steering Comittee. North American Symptomatic Carotid Surgery Trial**: Methods, patients, characteristics and progress. Stroke 22 (1991): 711-720

[2.3] **Barthels E**: Farbduplexsonographie der hirnversorgenden Gefäße. Atlas und Handbuch. Schattauer Verlag, Stuttgart, New York 194 (1999): 68

[2.4] **Widder B** : Doppler- und Duplexsonographie der hirnversorgenden Arterien. Springer-Verlag, Berlin, Heidelberg, 4. Aufl. (1995): 259-261

[2.5] **Fürst G, Saleh A, Wenserski F** et al: Reliability and validity of noninvasive imaging of internal carotid pseudo-occlusion. Stroke 30 (1999): 1444-1449

[2.6] **Sitzer M, Fürst G, Siebler M** et al: Usefulness of an intravenous contrast medium in the characterization of high-grade internal carotid stenosis with colour Doppler assisted duplex imaging. Stroke 25 (1994a): 385-389

[2.7] **Strandness DE, Eikelboom BC**: Carotid artery stenosis - where do we go from here? Eur J Ultrasound 7, Suppl 3 (1998): 17-26

[2.8] **Barthels E**: Duplexsonographie der Vertebralarterien, 1. Teil: Praktische Durchführung, Möglichkeiten und Grenzen der Methode, 2: Klinische Anwendungen. Ultraschall in Med 12 (1991): 54-69

[2.9] **Pignoli P, Tremoli E, Poli A,** et al: Intimal plus medial thickness of the arterial wall: a direct measurement with ultrasound imaging. Circulation 74 (1986): 1399-406.

[2.10] **Hodis HN, Mack WJ, LaBree L** et al: The role of carotid intima-media-thickness in predicting clinical coronary events. Ann Intern Med 128 (1998): 262-269.

[2.11] **Bots ML, Hoes AW, Koudstaal PJ** et al: Common carotid intima-media-thickness and risk of stroke and myocardial infarction. Circulation 96 (1997): 1432-1437.

[2.12] **Simon A, Gariepy J, Chironi G** et al: Intima- media thickness: a new tool for diagnosis and treatment of cardiovascular risk. J Hypertens 20 (2002): 159-169.

[2.13] **O´Leary DH, Polack JF, Kronmal RA, Manolio TA, Gregory LB, Wolfson SK**: Carotid- artery intima and media thickness as a risk factor for myocardial infarction and stroke in older adults. N Engl J Med 340 (1999): 14-22.

[2.14] **Sitzer M, Markus H, Medall M et al:** C reactive protein and carotid Intlma-media-thickness in a community population. J cardiovasc risk 2002; 9: 97-108

[2.15] **Hua Y, Meng XF, Jia LY et al.** Color Doppler imaging evaluation of proximal vertebral artery stenosis. American Journal of Radiology 193 (2009): 1434-1438

Chapter 3 / Thyroid

[3.1] **Castagnone D, Rivolta R, Rescalli S** et al: Color Doppler sonography in Graves disease: Value in assessing activity of disease and predicting outcome. ARJ 166 (1996): 203-207

[3.2] **Mende U, Zierhut D, Ewerbeck V** et al: Sonographische Kriterien für Staging und Verlaufskontrolle bei malignen Lymphonmen. Radiologie 37 (1997): 19-26

[3.3] **Na DG, Lim HK, Byun HS** et al: Differntial diagnosis of cervical lymphadenopathy: Usefulness of color doppler sonography. ARJ 168 (1997): 1311-1316

[3.4] **Saleh A, Santen R, Malms J** et al: B-Mode-Sonographie und moderne dopplersonographische Methoden bei Krankheiten der Schilddrüse und der Nebenschilddrüsen. Radiologe 38 (1998): 344-354

[3.5] **Steinkamp HJ, Cornehl M, Hosten N** et al: Cervial lymphadenopathy. Ratio of long-to-short-axsis diameter as a predictor of malignancy. Br.J.Radiol. 68 (1995): 266-270

[3.6] **Steinkamp HJ, Müffelmann M, Böck JC** et al: Diffrential diagnosis of lymph node lesions: a semiquantitative aproach with colour doppler ultrasound. Br.J.Radiol. 71 (1998): 823-833

Chapter 4 / Abdomen

[4.1] **Geelkerken RH, Lamers BHW** et al: Duodenal meal stimulation leads to coeliac artery vasoconstriction and superior mesenteric artery vasodilatation: an intraabdominal ultrasound study. Ultrasound in Med. 24, 9 (1998): 1351-56

[4.2] **Mirko P, Palazzoni A** et al: Sonographic and doppler assessment of the inrerior mesenteric artery: normal morphologic and hemodynamic features. Abdominal Imaging 23 (1998): 364-9

[4.3] **Geelkerken RH, Delahunt TA** et al: Pitfalls in the diagnosis of origin stenosis of the coeliac and superior mesenteric arteries with transabdominal color duplex examination. Ultrasound Med.Biol. 22, 6 (1996): 695-700

[4.4] **Perko MJ, Just S, Schroeder TV**: Importance of diastolic velocities in the detection of celiac and mesenteric artery disease by duplex ultrasound. J Vasc Surgery 26, 2 (1997): 288-93

[4.5] **Schuler A, Dirks K** et al: Das Ligamentum arcuatum-syndrom: Farbdopplersonographische Diagnose bei unklaren abdominalbeschwerden junger Patienten. Ultraschall in Med. 19 (1998): 157-163

[4.6] **Colli A, Coccioli M** et al: Abnormalities of Doppler waveform of the hepatic veins inpatients with chronic liver disease: Correlation with histological findings. AJR 162 (1994): 833-7

[4.7] **Helmberger T, Helmberger R** et al: Vena-Cava-Filter: Indikation, Komplikationen, Klinische Wertigkeit. Radiologe 38 (1998): 614-23

[4.8] **Hanisch E, Hebgen SO** et al: Zur Segmentanatomie der Leber – Eine sonomorphologische Sicht. Der Chirurg 70 (1990): 0169-73

[4.9] **Gallix BP, Taourel P** et al: Flow pulsantility in the portal venous system: a study of doppler sonography in healthy adults. AJR 169 (1997): 141-4

[4.10] **Fürst G, Malms J** et al: Transjugular intrahepatic portosystemic shunts: Improved evaluation with echo-enhanced color doppler sonography and spectral duplex sonography. AJR 170 (1998): 1047-54

[4.11] **Shapiro RS, Stancato-Pasik A** et al: Color doppler applications in hepatic imaging. Clinical Imaging 22 (1998): 272-9

[4.12] **Hosten N, Pils R** et al: Focal liver lesions: Doppler Ultrasound. Eur. Radiol. 9 (1999): 428-35

[4.13] **Gonzales-Anon M, Cervera-Dehal J** et al: Characterization of solid liver lesions with color and pulsed doppler imaging. Abdominal Imaging 24 (1999): 137-43

[4.14] **Leen E, Anderson JR** et al : Doppler index perfusion in the detection of herpatic metastases secondary to gastric carcinoma. Am.J.Surg. 173, 2 (1997): 99-102

[4.15] **Erden A, Cumhur T** et al: Superior mesenteric artery doppler waveform changes in response to inflammation of the ileocecal region. Abdominal Imaging 22 (1997): 483-6

[4.16] **Bunk A, Stoelben E** et al: Farbdopplerchirugie in der Leberchirugie. Ultraschall in Med. 19 (1998): 202-12

[4.17] **Kok T, Slooff MJH** et al: Routine doppler ultrasound for the detection of clinically unsuspected vascular complications in the early postoperative phase after orthotopic liever transplantation. Transpl. Int. 11 (1998): 272-6

[4.18] **Leen E**: The role of contrast-enhanced ultrasound in the characterization of focal liver lesions. Eur Radiol. 2001;11 Suppl 3:E27-34

[4.19] **Strobel D, Krodel U, Martus P** et al.: Clinical Evaluation of Contrast-Enhanced Color Doppler Sonography in the Differential Diagnosis of Liver Tumors. J Clin Ultrasound. 2000 Jan;28(1):1-13

[4.20] **Von Herbay A, Vogt C, Häussinger D**: Late-Phase Pulse-Inversion Sonography using the Contrast Agent Levovist: Differentiation beween benign and malignant focal lesions of the liver. AJR Am J Roentgenol. 2002 Nov;179(5):1273-9

[4.21] **Albrecht T, Blomley MJK, Burns PN** et al.: Improved Detection of Hepatic Metastases with Pulse-Inversion US during the Liver-Specific Phase of SHU 508A: A Multicenter Study. Radiology. 2003 May;227(2):361-70. Epub 2003 Mar 20

[4.22] **Hosten N, Puls R, Bechstein WO** et al.: Focal liver lesions: Doppler Ultrasound. Eur Radiol. 1999;9(3):428-35

[4.23] **Quaia E, Bertolotto M, Calderan L** et al. (2003): US characterization of focal hepatic lesions with intemittent high-acoustic-power Mode and Contrast Material. Acad Radiol. 2003 Jul;10(7):739-50

[4.24] **Krix M, Kiessling F, Hof H, Karcher A, Delorme S, Essig M** (2003): Liver Metastases show an homogenous arterial enhancement in intermittent low MI sonography using SonoVue. Abstract

Chapter 5 / Nephrology and urology

[5.1] **Krumme B, Kirschner T, Gondolf** et al: Altersabhänigkeit des intrarentalen Resistance Index (RI) bei essentiellen Hypertonikern. Bildgebung/Imaging (1994) Suppl. 2: 55

[5.2] **Krumme B, Blum U, Schwertfeger E** et al: Diagnosis of renovascular disease by intra- and extrarental Doppler scanning. Kidney int. 1996; 50: 1288-1292

[5.3] **Hollenbeck M, Kutkuhn B, Grabensee B:** Colour Dopler ultrasound in the diagnosis of transplant renal artery stenosis. Bildgebung/Imaging (1994) 61: 248-254

[5.4] **Rademacher J and Brunkhorst R:** Diagnosis and treatment of renovascular stenosis – a cost-benefit analysis. Nephrol. Dial.Transplant 1998 13: 2761-2767

[5.5] **Pickard RS, Oates CP, Sethia K** et al: The Role Colour Duplex Ultrasonography in the Diagnosis of Vasculogenic Impotence. Br.J.Urol. 68 (1991): 537-540

[5.6] **Chiou RK, Pomeroy BD, Chen WS** et al: Hermodynamic patterns of pharmacologically induced erection: Evaluation by color doppler sonographpy J.Urol. 159 (1998): 109-112

[5.7] **Meulemann EJH, Bemelmans BLH, van Asten WN** et al: Assement of penile blood flow by duplex ultrasonography in 44 men with normal erectile potency in different phases of erection. J.Urol. 147 (1992): 51-55

[5.8] **Kadioglu A, Erdogru T, Karsidag K** et al: Evaluation of Penile Arterial System with Color Doppler Ultrasonography in Nondiabetic and Diabetic Males. Euro. Urol. 27 (1995): 311-314

[5.9] **Schwartz AN, Wang KY, Mach LA** et al: Evaluation of normal erectiel function with color flow doppler sonography. ARJ 153 (1989): 1155-1160

[5.10] **Porst H:** Die Duplexsonographie des Penis. Urologie [A] 32 (1993): 242-249

[5.11] **Fürst G, Müller-Mattheis V, Cohnen M** et al: Venous incompetence in erectile dysfunction: Evaluation with color-coded duplex sonography and cavernosometry/-graphy. Eur. Radiology 9 (1999): 35-41

[5.12] **Chiou RK, Anderson JC, Chen WS** et al: Hemodynamic evaluation of erectile dysfunction and Peyronie´s Diseases using color doppler ultrasound. J.US Med. 16 (1997): 20-24

[5.13] **Sanders LM, Haber S, Dembner A** et al: Significane of reversal of diastloic flow in the acute scrotum. J.US Med. 16 (1997): 20-24

[5.14] **Luker GD, Siegel MJ:** Color Doppler Sonography of the Scrotum in Children. AJR 163 (1994): 649-655

[5.15] **Berman JM, Beidle TR, Kunberger LE** et al: Sonographic Evaluation of Acute Intrascrotal Pathology. AJR. 166 (1996): 857-861

[5.16] **Herbener TE:** Ultrasound in the Assessment of the Acute Scrotum. J. Clin Ultrasound 24 (1996): 405-421

[5.17] **Becker D, Bürst M, Wehler M** et al: Differnetialdiagnose des Hodenschmerzes mit der farbkodierten Duplexsonographie. Dtsch. Med Wschr. 122 (1997): 1405-1409

[5.18] **Özcan H, Aytac S, Yagi C** et al: Color Doppler Ultrasonographic Findings in Intratesticular Varicocele. Clin Ultrasound 25 (1997): 325-329

[5.19] **Lehmann K, Kacl G, Hagspiel K** et al: Die Wertigkeit der farbkodierten Duplexsonographie als Standardabklärung bei erektiler Dysfunktion. Urologe [A] 35 (1996): 456-462

[5.20] **Radermacher J, Chavan A, Bleck J,** et al.: Use of Doppler ultrasonography to predict the outcome of therapy for renal-artery stenosis. N Engl J Med. 2001; 344: 410-417

[5.21] **Sands J, Miranda C:** Prolongation of hemodialysis access survival with elective revision. Clin-Nephrol. 44 (1995): 329-333

[5.22] **Stavros AT, Parker SH, Yakes WF** et al: Segmental stenosis of the renal artery: pattern recognition of tardus and parvus abnormalities with duplex sonography. Radiology 184 (1992): 487-492

Chapter 6 / Obstetrics and gynecology

[6.1] **AIUM Bioeffects commitee:** Bioeffects considerations for safety in ultrasound. J.Ultrasound Med. Suppl.7 (1988): 1-38

[6.2] **Maulik D:** Doppler Ultrasound in Obstetrics & Gynacology. Springer Verlag New York, Berlin, Heidelberg. (1977)

[6.3] **Sohn C, Holzgreve W:** Ultraschall in Gynäkologie und Geburtshilfe.Georg Thieme Verlag Stuttgart, London. (1995): 501-540

[6.5] **Carter J, Perrone T, Carson LF** et al: Uterine malignancy predictid by transvaginal sonography and color flow doppler ultrasonography. J Clin Ultrasound 21 (1993): 405-408

[6.6] **Steer CV, Millis CL, Campbell S:** Vaginal color doppler assement on the day of embryo transfer (ET) accurately predicts patients in an in-vitro fertilisation programme with suboptimal uterine perfusion who fail to become pregnant. Ultrasound Obstet Gynecol 1 (1991): 79

[6.7] **Vetter K:** Dopplersonographie in der Schwangerschaft. VHC, Weinheim (1991)

[6.8] **Kurjak A, Zalud I, Alfirevic Z:** Evaluation of adnexal masses with transvaginal color ultrasound. J Ultrasound Med 10 (1991): 295-299.

[6.9] **Laurin J, Marschal K, Persson PH** et al: Ultrasound measurement of the fetal blood flow in predicting fetal outcome. Br J Obstet Gynecol 94 (1987): 940-948

[6.10] **Indik JH, Chen V, Reed KL :** Assosiation of umbilical venous with inferior vena cava blood Flow velocities. Obstet Gynecol 77 (1991): 551-557

[6.11] **Hucke J:** Extrauteringravidität: klinisches Bild, Diagnostik, Therapie und spätere Fertilität. Wiss. Verl.-Ges., Stuttgart (1997)

[6.12] **Taylor KJW, Ramos IM, Feyock A** et al: Ectopic Pregnancy: duplex Doppler evaluation. Radiology 173 (1998): 93-96

[6.13] **Lindner C, Hünecke B, Schlotfeld T** et al : Vaginale Kontrastmittelsonographie zur Prüfung der Tubendurchgängigkeit. Fertilität 5 (1989): 173-178

[6.14] **Alle Normkurven aus PIA-Fetal Database (1998)**

Chapter 7 / Peripheral arteries

[7.1] **Wolf KJ, Fobbe F:** Farbkodierte Duplexsonographie. Grundlagen und klinische Anwendung. Georg Thieme Verlag, Stuttgart, New York (1993): 125

[7.2] **Reimer P, Landwehr P:** Non-invasive vascular imaging of peripheral vessels, Eur. Radiology 8; 6 (1998): 858-872

[7.3] **Heintzen HP, Strauer BE:** Periphere arterielle Komplikationen nach Herzkatheteruntersuchungen. Herz 23 (1998): 4-20

[7.4] **Ugurluoglu A, Katzenschlager R** et al: Ultrasound guided compression therapy in 134 patients with iatrogenic pseudo-aneurysms: advantage of routine douplex ultrasound control of the punkture site following transfemoral catheterization. VASA 26 (1997): 110-116

[7.5] **Beissert M, Jenett M, Kellner M** et al: Panoramabildverfahren SieScape in der radiologischen Diagnostik. Radiologe 38 (1998): 410-416

[7.6] **Sacks D, Robinson ML, Marinelli DL** et al: Peripheral arterial Doppler ultrasonography: diagnostic criteria. J.US. Med 11; 3 (1992): 95-103

[7.7] **Treiman GS, Lawrence PF, Galt SW** et al: Revision of revesed infrainguinal bypass grafts without preoperativ arteriography. J.Vasc.Surg 26; 6 (1997): 1020-8

[7.8] **Chatterjee T, Do DD, Mahler F** et al: Pseudoaneurysm of femoral artery after catheterisation: treatment by a mechanical compression device guided by colour Doppler ultrasound. Heart 79; 5 (1998): 502-4

[7.9] **Sands J, Miranda C:** Prolongation of hemodialysis acces survival with elective revision. Clin-Nephrol. 44 (1995): 329-33

[7.10] **Sands JJ, Kapsick B, Brinckman M:** Assessment of hemodialysis access performance by color-flow Doppler ultrasound. J Biometer Appl 13 (1999): 224-237

Chapter 8 / Peripheral veins

[8.1] **Bernadi E, Camporese G, Büller HR et al.** Serial 2-Point Ulrasonography plus D-Dimer vs. whleleg Color-Coded Doppler Ultrasonography for diagnosing suspected symptomatic deep vein thrombosis. JAMA 2008; 300 (14): 1653-1659

[8.2] **Dauzat M, Laroche JP, Deklunder G** et al: Diagnosos of acute limb deep venous thrombosis with ultrasound: trends and controversies. J.Clin. Ultrasound 25 (1997): 343-358

[8.3] **Fraser JD, Anderson DR:** Deep venous thrombosis: recent advances and optimal investigation with US. Radiology 211(1999): 9-24

Chapter 9 / Echocardiography

[9.1] **Feigenbaum, Harvey:** Echocardiography, 5th ed., Lea & Febiger, Philadelphia (1994)

[9.2] **Köhler, Eckehard:** Klinische Echokardiographie, Enke, Stuttgart, (1996)

[9.3] **Hatle, Liv:** Doppler ultrasound in cardiology, 2nd ed., Lea & Febiger, Philadelphia (1985)

[9.4] **Kruck I, Biamino G:** Quantitative Methoden der M-Mode-, 2D- und Doppler-Echokardiographie, Böhringer, Mannheim (1988)

[9.5] **Moltzahn S, Zeydabadinejad M:** Doppler-Echokardiographie Thieme, Stuttgard (1995)

[9.6] **Moltzahn S:** Ein- und Zweidimensionale Echokardiographie, Thieme, Stuttgart (1992)

Chapter 10 / Technical innovations

[10.1] **Baulmann J, Nürnberger J, Slany J** et al. Arterial stiffness and pulse wave analysis: consensus paper on basics, methods and clinical applications. Dtsch Med Wochenschr 2010; 135: 4-14

[10.2] **Laurent S, Cockroft J, Van Bortel L** et al. Expert consensus document on arterial stiffness: methodological issues and clinical applications. European Heart Journal 2006; 27: 2588-2605